Understanding
Postpartum Psychosis

Understanding Postpartum Psychosis

A Temporary Madness

Teresa M. Twomey, JD

with Shoshana Bennett, PhD

Foreword by Katherine Wisner, MD, MS

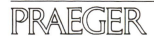

Westport, Connecticut
London

Library of Congress Cataloging-in-Publication Data

Twomey, Teresa M., 1965-
    Understanding postpartum psychosis : a temporary
madness / Teresa M. Twomey
with Shoshana Bennett ; foreword by Katherine Wisner.
        p. cm.
    Includes bibliographical references and index.
    ISBN 978-0-313-35346-8 (alk. paper)
1. Motherhood. 2. Postpartum depression. I. Title.
    HQ759.T96   2009
    618.7′6—dc22   2008046272

British Library Cataloguing in Publication Data is available.

Library of Congress Catalog Card Number: 2008046272
ISBN: 978-0-313-35346-8

First published in 2009

Praeger Publishers, 88 Post Road West, Westport, CT 06881
An imprint of Greenwood Publishing Group, Inc.
www.praeger.com

Printed in the United States of America

∞

The paper used in this book complies with the
Permanent Paper Standard issued by the National
Information Standards Organization (Z39.48-1984).

10 9 8 7 6 5 4 3 2 1

This book contains research and ideas of the authors but is not, in any way,
intended as medical or legal advice or as a substitute for medical or legal
advice. PPP is a serious illness which requires immediate medical attention by
a mental health or medical professional. The authors and publisher disclaim
any liability from any adverse affects connected to or arising from, directly or
indirectly, any information or opinion contained in this book.

To my daughters, especially Ariana

Contents

Foreword

I met Teresa a few years ago at a meeting convened by the National Institute of Mental Health for the purpose of federal grant evaluations. She was impressive as a reviewer who represented the interests and views of the public. Her astute comments and competent interpersonal style drew me to know more about her. When she told me she had experienced postpartum psychosis, my immediate response was that she was an incredible model of recovery for women and families. Teresa joins a cadre of women, health care professionals, celebrities, and politicians in revealing the impact of postpartum psychiatric morbidity. At a time when society expects a beaming, well-coiffed new mother with a beautiful rosy-cheeked baby in a clean outfit, the mother with psychosis cannot organize her own care much less that of her infant. The fundamental sense of self that defines us all is fractured for her. I was impressed with Teresa's comment to me in an email: "My goal is simply to help women who have or will suffer postpartum psychosis. Anything you might have to say would be received by me in the spirit of someone who is also concerned for these women and their families."

As former Surgeon General David Satcher proclaimed, mental health is fundamental to health. Women are the most vulnerable to psychosis in the post-birth period than at any other time during their lives. In the first thirty days after birth, a woman is more than twenty times as likely to develop psychosis than in the two-year period prior to childbirth. If she has not had a child before, she is thirty-five times more likely to suffer psychosis than women with children. About 1–2 per 1000 new mothers suffer psychosis and 1 of 7 develops depression, with a similar number becoming depressed during pregnancy. Clearly, postpartum psychiatric disorders are a major public health concern.

Our societal question is: Why have we not implemented universal mental health screening for pregnant and postpartum women? Screening measures exist, effective treatment is available, and intervention holds the promise of improving the entire family's (and more broadly the community's) well being. There is political action in the MOTHERS Act (Mom's Opportunity to Access Help, Education, Research, and Support for Postpartum Depression), passed overwhelmingly in the U.S. House of Representatives on October 15, 2007 and pending in the U.S. Senate as of June 15, 2008, which has raised awareness and impacted public policy.

In vulnerable women, the brain is differentially sensitive to the massive withdrawal of hormones that occurs at delivery. The reasons for the vulnerability of postpartum women to mental illness and the pathophysiology related to post-birth disorders are the subject of international investigation. Sleep deprivation and marked interference with circadian rhythms related to labor are likely contributors to mood instability. The clinical picture of postpartum psychosis is characterized by rapid onset of hectic mood fluctuation, marked cognitive impairment suggestive of delirium, bizarre behavior, insomnia, visual and auditory hallucinations, and unusual hallucinations (tactile and olfactory). My research team found that postpartum psychosis is frequently a manifestation of bipolar illness: mania and/or depression with psychotic features. Women with acute onset psychoses related to childbearing usually experienced recurrence of previously undiagnosed cyclical mood disorders rather than the triggering of a new disorder. The implication is that careful screening during childbearing holds promise for early identification or preventive treatment.

Prevention of infanticide, an associated tragedy of psychosis, involves increased awareness and a heightened index of suspicion by all health care professionals, patients, and their families. Women with a previous episode of postpartum psychosis and women with bipolar disorder are at high risk for postpartum mental illness. Why wait? Postpartum monitoring for the emergence of symptoms should be a collaborative plan between the physician and the patient's family. Preventive medication at birth or rapid, pre-determined medication initiation for women who develop symptoms, with a family monitoring plan for the infant for safety while the mother recovers, are crucial. Psychosocial therapies help the woman and her family understand the illness and treatment approach. Behavioral techniques that target daily rhythms help patients regularize their routines, diminish interpersonal problems, adhere to medication regimes, and improve function.

As I write this foreword, I am recalling the early days of my medical career in the mid-1980s. I remember heated debates with colleagues who claimed: "There is no such thing as postpartum psychosis—it's not in the Diagnostic and Statistical Manual" (the diagnostic manual for mental illnesses), "Postpartum disorders are specific to that time; if a woman doesn't have another baby she won't get sick again," "Women are fulfilled during pregnancy so they don't become mentally ill," or the contradicting, "You can't prescribe medication for a woman who is pregnant or breastfeeding." How incredulous these statements seem from this vantage point twenty plus years later. I truly hope the pace of discovery accelerates on behalf of childbearing women and some other investigator can be even more incredulous in another twenty years.

Katherine Wisner, MD, MS
Professor of Psychiatry, Obstetrics and Gynecology
and Reproductive Sciences, Epidemiology
and Women's Studies
Director, Women's Behavioral HealthCARE
University of Pittsburgh, Pittsburgh, PA

Acknowledgments

First and foremost I thank all the women who have written and trusted me with their stories, those that appear in this book and those that do not. All have informed my understanding. To all of you: your trust, honesty, and passion to help others who have suffered or will suffer are astonishing.

Second, I thank my husband, Drew, for being my biggest cheerleader, Mr. Mom, and loving partner, and without whose moral and financial support this book would not be possible. Along with him I thank my children, who probably do not remember a time before I began this book. They have grown to show incredible maturity and generosity when I was working on the book or taking a call from a woman in need.

A big Thank You: To Jane Honikman, who encouraged me from the start. To my brother, Mike Twomey, for his generosity in being my graphic designer and "webmaster," and my brother, Luke Twomey, who helped me with the formatting of this book. To all of those who helped to type, review, and edit my rough drafts, particularly Deb Kaszas, Molly Preudhomme, Rosemarie Twomey, and Drew Harris. I also thank Elizabeth Peters, who helped me with the citations and bibliography.

To my mom, Rosemarie Twomey, who edited and listened and encouraged me to write this book, and to my father, Daniel Twomey, whose support was unwavering. It is difficult to write something that can cast loved-ones in a bad light. There is no blame or shame due to any of my family members for their actions or inactions. When I began giving talks about my experience, audience members often expressed their anger at my husband and my parents. That anger is misplaced. I've not been an easy person to live with—as a daughter or a wife—and the fault is not theirs.

Thank you to all the members of my Discipleship class for their early encouragement and support.

During my postpartum period I was desperate for help. For those who came to my aid, especially Lauren Sutter Jones, Joanne Mixen, Judy and Noel Kropf, Mike Twomey, and Edna Rockwell Harris, I thank you. You may have helped to save my life; you certainly helped me regain sanity. I know there were *many* more who would have come if they had *any* idea how bad it was, but you were the ones who came anyway.

A huge thank you to Dr. Shoshana Bennett for agreeing to write the first two chapters of this book. Her experience, expertise, and accessible writing style have made this a much better book. Dr. Shosh has been a mentor and friend, and as much as I wish I'd known her while I was going through my postpartum experience, I am grateful for her role in my healing process.

To all who allowed me to interview them, notably Dr. Margaret Spinelli, and George Parnham, J.D. To all who contributed items, notably Lauren Hale and Cheryl Jazzar. To Wendy Davis and Devani Stumpf for digging up and compiling historical information on PSI. Many people have offered encouragement, support, and opportunities to further this project; although you are too many to list, I thank you all. I also thank Stan Wakefield, who found a publisher for me in an amazingly short period of time, and Debra Carvalko at Praeger/Greenwood who offered advice and suggestions that undoubtedly have made this a better book. And, of course, I thank all those at Praeger/Greenwood who believed in the importance of this topic.

Introduction

"Saving the lives of babies and mothers." That's the short answer to why I began to write this book. In the Harry Potter stories, "the wand ... chooses the wizard."[1] In this case I feel "the book chose the author." It began with recognition of one need, but as it evolved, I realized there are many levels of need for many people regarding this illness.

USE OF THE TERM "POSTPARTUM PSYCHOSIS"

In recent years, postpartum disorders with distinct characteristics such as postpartum obsessive-compulsive disorder and postpartum post-traumatic stress disorder have been identified and have called for different screening and treatment protocols. I think in the future, different types of psychosis with distinct characteristics may be identified as well. For example, a psychosis with an underlying schizophrenia may require different treatment than a psychosis that is triggered by dehydration, bipolar disorder or by a thyroid disorder. I expect this would indicate different treatment protocols and predict different rates of recurrence. However, because such distinctions are not yet part of the general discourse, this book will simply refer to postpartum psychosis as a singular disorder.

RECOGNITION

PPP (postpartum psychosis) was the worse experience of my life. But I was lucky; no one was physically hurt, and both my child and my marriage survived. And I do mean *lucky*! I was not diagnosed or treated. But still I lost much. I lost the joy of new motherhood. I lost "me" for the first two years of my daughter's life. It was almost two years before I learned the name for my experience and even longer to put the pieces together. So you might imagine my anger when I first discovered that with proper screening, this illness is *preventable*, and when it is not prevented, it is very *treatable*. But because medical professionals cannot agree about whether this is a distinct illness or simply one that manifests itself postpartum, there is no independent diagnostic code, no standard screening, no standards of treatment.

There is no question that the women who suffer this illness are severely mentally ill. The issue is what to call this illness and whether it calls for a distinct official diagnosis. Currently it is treated as falling within one of three categories of mental illness, but does not have a separate diagnosis. One problem is that the symptoms of PPP do not neatly fall into any one particular category, and a woman may have symptoms of all three of these categories at once. To reconcile this, women with this illness are generally diagnosed with whichever illness their symptoms most closely resemble and then are treated accordingly. That might not pose a problem, except for the fact that, in reality, this has led to the perception among the uninformed that this illness does not actually exist. To be clear—the illness exists. The terminology—what it is called, *if* it has any specific name, if it should be a distinct diagnosis—is at issue.

Some experts believe that what we call "postpartum psychosis" is simply the exacerbation of pre-existing, but perhaps undiagnosed, cyclical mood disorders. Whether or not that is the case, our current practice regarding women with this illness is clearly insufficient. Women are still undiagnosed, misdiagnosed, and insufficiently treated.

Ironically, if PPP *is* the result of a pre-existing condition, the *good news* is that we have the technology *now* to accurately screen for this illness and take action to prevent it. However, because we wait until a crisis prompts treatment for mental illness, and because a substantial percentage of women have this crisis in the postpartum period, we continue to miss these opportunities for prevention. The significance of the postpartum period has been so overlooked that even women with a previous diagnosis do not always receive preventative treatment. However, even *if* this illness had *no* biochemical relationship to childbirth, other aspects of the postpartum period justify additional attention to the risk of mental illness postpartum.

We know that a postpartum woman is probably caring for at least one child—an infant. We know that many of the ordinary aspects of the postpartum period—moodiness, disrupted sleep, difficulty thinking clearly, changes in behavior and habits—can mask the symptoms of mental illness. We know that certain factors, such as loss of sleep, can exacerbate mental illness. Furthermore, our societal myths of motherhood provide incentive for women to hide their symptoms if or when they can *and* may lead others to dismiss statements these women make that in other contexts would clearly indicate a problem.

We also know that there are other potential physical complications that may contribute to mood problems—from difficult physical recoveries, to hormonal changes, to thyroid and pituitary problems. And we know that many women face relative isolation following the birth of a child. Therefore, they are likely to have less exposure to those who might notice changes that would indicate the onset of a mental illness.

However, because there is no official diagnosis or recognition of postpartum vulnerabilities, women and their families remain uninformed, providers are not trained, preventative measures remain ignored, missed diagnoses and misdiagnoses remain common, and suffering continues. I can only imagine the bitterness of those who have lost their children because of this. If official recognition is necessary for adequate treatment, then we need official recognition of this disorder *now*. If things remain as they are, we can be certain more preventable tragedies will occur, and babies and their mothers will die.

EDUCATION

After Andrea Yates drowned her children in Texas, the comments I heard convinced me that there is a huge gulf between common beliefs and the realities of mental illness. When my laid-back younger brother, who I'd never heard say a bad word about anyone, startled me with his reaction to news about Andrea Yates by saying, "Women like that should burn in hell!," I knew I needed to do something to educate people about this illness. I started right then with my brother, telling him that I could have been like Andrea Yates.

Around that same time I was praying for guidance about my life, asking, "What should I do with my life, my career?" Over and over I felt called to write this book, *immediately*. For months I resisted the idea—I had three children under the age of four—*and* I feared the stigma associated with mental illness. I feared meeting strangers who might know intimate details of my life. I still do. But my conviction eventually became stronger than my fears. I called Jane Honikman to ask permission to request stories from members of Postpartum Support International. She was very encouraging. At first I asked for stories across the spectrum of postpartum mood disorders because I did not believe I could gather enough PPP stories to make a book. I was wrong. Not only did I collect enough stories for my book, but most of the contributors were willing to use their real names! (I've decided against using real names because of logistical complications regarding publisher requirements.)

HEALING

Each story taught me something and each made me cry. And each one helped me heal a little bit more. In fact, the more stories I read, the more I was convinced of the need for this book. I realized this was needed for more than educating others. It was needed so that women who have had this illness, and their families, can read the stories of others to facilitate their own healing. There is nothing like reading or hearing these stories to fully understand "It's not just me!" It is important to realize there are two levels of recovery from this illness. There is recovery from the biochemical illness itself, and there is post-recovery recovery from having had the illness: the healing of psyche, ego, self-esteem, confidence, and relationships. I have been so impressed with the healing power of these stories that this possibility of healing has become my primary motivation for writing this book.

It is not just the women who have suffered who need to know that they are not alone. The families and spouses also need to know that they are not alone, and that the illness is not permanent. This illness kills marriages and injures relationships. Hurtful things may have been done or said. And all members of the family may need to learn to trust again. Understanding this illness can greatly facilitate that healing.

The women who sent me their stories are neither saints nor freaks. They represent all of womankind—wealthy and poor, in bad situations and ideal situations, some with a history of mental illness, and others with no history of it. Most are married, but not all of them. For some this illness struck with their first child, for some it was a subsequent birth. The experience was traumatic even for those who recovered without incident.

PREVENTION

I then spent years looking for a publisher. There were plenty of times I wanted to give up or became busy with some other project, but then I would hear of yet another tragedy and feel like I should have had this book out yesterday. We *must* do more to prevent these tragedies. We have some of the tools; we need the will to apply them. We know that taking more detailed histories can better identify those with higher risk factors. When risk is known, some professionals have been successful in preventing the illness itself (see Sichel and Driscoll, and Hamilton, in Appendix A). I believe that with more research and educated professionals, we may actually eradicate this illness!

When this illness is not prevented, early screening may uncover indications of postpartum psychosis and allow for early intervention. This is important because of the rapid onset and waxing and waning aspects of this illness. Family members who are aware of the symptoms and risks of this illness are more likely to respond quickly and effectively. Medical providers on all levels—from the delivery floor or general practitioner to the paramedic or emergency room worker—must know how to identify these women and respond appropriately.

The stories in this book can help to dispel the myths about what we expect from this illness and help the reader understand and recognize the warning signs.

REFORM

Take a moment and consider: "Which group of medical professionals who deal with pregnant and postpartum women take upon themselves the responsibility to evaluate the women's mental health?" The family practitioner, who might know the woman best, is largely replaced by the obstetrician-gynecologist (OB-GYN) during this period. The OB-GYNs, as a profession, have not claimed responsibility for evaluating whether a woman may have a mental health issue; their concern is the physical outcome of the pregnancy and the health of the infant. The nurses and midwives often lack the specific training or mandate to evaluate a woman's mental health. The pediatrician is the health professional the woman likely sees more than any other after the birth of her baby, but the woman is not a patient of the pediatrician. So the responsibility to identify a mental health issue in a postpartum woman generally falls on her and her family—those *least* qualified to do so. When onset is rapid and severe, prompt diagnosis can be critical. It seems absurd to count on laypersons for this. Where the woman has no history of mental illness, the family may be in denial or may confuse her symptoms with ordinary postpartum adjustment. Normal women do not go into pregnancy thinking they will become psychotic, or even homicidal. Nor do their families expect this. We need better communication among medical professionals, and we need them to step up to the plate and take responsibility for the mental health assessment of pregnant and postpartum women.

The reform of our legal system, in relationship to this illness, is necessary for basic fairness and humane treatment for these women—two central tenets of care in a "civilized" society. My concern with both the medical and the legal treatment of women with PPP is also personal for me. Along the way I learned that this illness may sometimes have hereditary components (just as bipolar disorder and schizophrenia may have hereditary components). In fact, recent research indicates a genetic cause. I have three daughters. So, another purpose for this book is to effect change in the medical field so the steps and procedures necessary to prevent this illness are in place by the time my daughters have children. I don't want them to face doctors who deny the reality of this illness. Most of all, I don't want my daughters to go through what the women of this book have—not when it is *preventable*!

If preventative measures are not in place and tragedy strikes my family, I would want my child to be treated with dignity and compassion by all involved. I would want her to receive the best legal representation possible, which means defense attorneys who are willing to take on such a case and who are educated about this illness. I would want a legal system that recognizes the unique qualities of this tragic illness. I would not want to lose my daughter to death or prison.

LOOKING FOR ANSWERS

There is still much that we don't know, and much that needs to be done. Although I have managed to help many women and families through peer support, there are *more* that I have not been able to help. It is heartbreaking to not have the answers. I've been asked by women and families in crisis: "Where can we get adequate treatment for my daughter? We've been to three hospitals. Money is no object!"; "Will my insurance cover it, and if it doesn't where do I go?"; "Why does my wife hate me?"; "What can I do to get my wife back (to help her become well) when all she does is fight me?"; "She won't even speak to me—what do I do?"; "How can we persuade her to take the treatments?"

Too many times I've cried when I've hung up the phone. Too many times I've worried about what I might see on the news. We need more research, more understanding and procedures for intervention, more knowledge of what helps and what exacerbates this illness, more ways to identify those at risk and to gauge the level of risk, more certainty regarding causes and treatment, and *standard procedures* for prevention. Although I'm happy to help, those in crisis need better resources than a volunteer layperson on the telephone! I want this book to inspire researchers, legal and medical professionals, our public servants, and our communities to actively seek answers to these questions.

COMMUNITY INVOLVEMENT

Finally, we need to understand that this illness can, in one way or another, affect any of us. We need education of the community. We need a community of support for new mothers. Babies are the most vulnerable and helpless members of our society. Mothers with severe mental illness are also vulnerable and helpless members of our society. In some ways it is surprising that over 90 percent of these women *do not* harm anyone. Yet, we continue to act shocked when tragedy occurs when these ill women are left to care for babies.

Most people I speak to about this illness fall into one of four categories: those who know that they or a member of their family is at risk and want to learn as much as possible; those who are curious but do not believe this illness could touch their family; those who *formerly* did not think this illness could touch their family (or did not know of this illness) who say, "If we'd only known . . ."; and those who continue to deny the existence of this illness. When this illness happens to the unsuspecting woman, unnecessary suffering is almost guaranteed. It is only by educating the whole community, whether its members think this applies to them or not, that we can really hope to prevent this illness and its associated tragedies.

The good news about education on this topic is that the central message is not one of *fear* but is one of *hope*! The women who suffer this are not alone (this illness occurs at the same rate as Down Syndrome); they are not to blame (this is not a choice they make but is biochemical); there is *help* (there are treatments to *prevent* this illness and treatments to *cure* this illness); and for the vast majority of sufferers, with appropriate care *they will be well.*

WARNING TO WOMEN WITH POSTPARTUM OBSESSIVE-COMPULSIVE DISORDER

Women with postpartum OCD (obsessive-compulsive disorder)—having intrusive and disturbing thoughts, sometimes about harming their child—are advised NOT to read the first-person stories until after they have recovered. Women with OCD often "borrow" from others' intrusive thoughts—that is, they read or hear of someone else's intrusive thoughts and then they start having those thoughts as well. If you suspect you have OCD, speak to your medical professional about this and, if necessary, receive treatment before reading any of the stories in this book!

Furthermore, this book contains some graphic and disturbing descriptions of mental illness. Women with PPMDs or who are just beginning their recovery may want to skip parts or wait until they are further along in their recovery to read this book. However, I have been told by women who *have* fully recovered from PPMDs, particularly psychosis, that hearing my story or reading one of these stories was healing in a way that nothing else had been.

HOW THIS BOOK IS ORGANIZED

The first section of this book provides a broad overview to assist the reader in understanding this illness. The first two chapters give the medical perspective and distinguish between PPP and postpartum OCD, which can appear similar but are quite different in terms of treatment and risks. Chapters three and four address how this illness is treated in historical accounts, modern media, and our legal system. These demonstrate how the current approach compounds the suffering of and even re-victimizes women with this illness and offer suggestions for change.

The second section of this book contains first-person stories of PPP. With one exception (the suicide), these were written by the women who suffered this illness. Their accounts have received minimal editing to preserve the authentic "voice" of these women. All generously offered their stories in order to help other women. They did not receive any compensation for their contributions. I made the choice to use fictional names although most of the women were willing to allow me to use their real names. (There are two exceptions to this as those two stories are already public in one form or another.) Using the real names of my contributors would do little to add to the many sources available to establish the veracity of the illness and types of symptoms. The primary purpose of this book is to educate, heal, and call for change.

I deliberately chose to include only one suicide and one infanticide story. The remaining are stories of recovery. I did this because the vast majority of women who suffer this illness recover without hurting anyone, but they are largely in hiding—both historically and in present-day society.

Because these are personal, unfiltered stories, they are likely to include the author's views, opinions, and judgments about her subjective experience, and they should be understood as such. At times some may be confusing or hard to follow. You may want to consider that such a reaction is more indicative of our expectation of clarity and is not something that needs to be "fixed." You might consider that these stories are as close as most of you will come to experiencing psychosis from the inside. They also provide the graphic grounding of the descriptions of psychosis and OCD provided in chapters one and two. The reader may want to alternate reading and re-reading chapters one and two and the stories.

The book concludes with a call for action in the chapter, "What We Know, Don't Know, and Need to Do to Prevent Tragedy." Appendixes A and B then provide resources for further reading and where to find help.

List of Abbreviations

DM	(*Dangerous Motherhood*)
DSM	(*Diagnostic and Statistical Manual of Mental Disorders*)
DSM-IV	(*Diagnostic and Statistical Manual of Mental Disorders*, 4th Edition)
ECT	(electroconvulsive therapy)
ER	(emergency room)
ICU	(intensive care unit)
IV	(intravenous)
MPC	(Model Penal Code)
OB	(obstetrician)
OB-GYN	(obstetrician/gynecologist)
OCD	(obsessive-compulsive disorder)
PMDs	(postpartum mood disorders)
PMS	(premenstrual syndrome)
PP	(postpartum)
PPD	(postpartum depression)
PPMD	(postpartum mood disorder)
PPP	(postpartum psychosis)
PSI	(Postpartum Support International)
SIDS	(sudden infant death syndrome)
UPP	(*Understanding Postpartum Psychosis*)

PART I

Overview

To fully understand this illness and to serve as an advocate for the women who suffer this illness—as a spouse, as a family member, as a medical provider, as an attorney, as a concerned member of the public, or even as an advocate for yourself—it is helpful to understand the context in which this illness occurs.

One of the central issues regarding this illness is recognition. Currently there is insufficient recognition of this illness. It is not recognized as an official medical diagnosis. It is not recognized by mainstream books on women, history, and madness. It is often incorrectly described by contemporary media. And it is not recognized as a distinct illness by the legal system.

The first chapter of this book, by Dr. Shoshana Bennett, an expert on postpartum mood disorders, distinguishes between different types of mood disorders. Because this illness is often misidentified, she illustrates what it is and what it is not. It is not depression. Women who have terrible thoughts about hurting their children are often diagnosed as psychotic but they are *not*.

In the next chapter, Bennett describes the medical view and illustrates the unique features of this illness. She addresses risk analysis, treatment, and prevention. Ideally these chapters would be general knowledge among all practitioners who interact with and treat perinatal and postpartum women. Current standard training does not cover symptoms of this as a distinct disorder because it is not *recognized* as a distinct disorder. Therefore most of the professionals with whom a postpartum woman interacts may not have adequate training to notice symptoms that would indicate a disorder and, significantly, may not appreciate the level of risk associated with those symptoms. And most spouses and family members are equally unaware and uninformed.

Our cultural dialogue does little to inform the general public that ordinary women—women who function well domestically and professionally, who do not suspect themselves and whose family and friends do not suspect of having a mental disorder—could become so mentally ill after having a baby that they actually become *psychotic*, that they might even become *homicidal*. And our cultural dialogue does even less to reassure those women and their families that most of these women recover completely and quickly without harming anyone. As the third chapter shows, the common features of this illness, the naming of this illness, and even the connection between childbirth and subsequent mental illness, are largely absent from popular discourse on women, madness, and infanticide. True, media accounts that name this illness and link childbirth and subsequent mental illness are becoming more common. But they are often inaccurate and misleading.

The lack of official recognition contributes to a number of problems. The first is that medical providers do not screen "ordinary women" for this disorder, and opportunities for the prevention of the illness are missed. The second is that when it does occur, both the woman's medical personnel and her family do not recognize her behavior as indicative of a problem, and opportunities for prompt, effective treatment are missed. The third is that when this illness causes behavior that results in death or injury to the woman or others, lack of recognition by the medical community leads to the lack of recognition by the legal community. Because the legal community heavily relies on *evidence* and *inference*, it looks to official medical standards and diagnoses and what can be inferred from those. Where there is no distinct DSM diagnosis, the symptoms a woman may have experienced that did not fit into her "official diagnosis" are extremely difficult to prove. Not only are they not inferred from the diagnosis, but it might be implied that they were absent because they are not typically present in that particular disorder. Therefore this lack of recognition leads to a number of interconnected problems that these women face when confronted by the legal system in the United States. Although there are a number of legal issues that can arise from this disorder, this book utilizes infanticide to illustrate the "perfect storm" these women face. The chapter on law includes practical suggestions for attorneys who represent these women and information on legislation.

In providing the societal context of this illness, this section highlights the many problems lack of recognition can cause. It is my belief that denying something a name often serves to deny its very existence. How do we discuss something that lacks a name? How do we guard against it? How can it be explained it to others? How do those who have suffered know they have recovered? Recognition is not a panacea, but lack of recognition unnecessarily creates a complicated web of problems that contribute to the suffering, tragedy, and injustices these women and their families face.

Chapter 1

More than Depression: Differences Among Postpartum Psychosis, Postpartum Depression, and Postpartum Obsessive-Compulsive Disorder

Shoshana Bennett, PhD

Postpartum mood and anxiety disorders affect hundreds of thousands of women every year in the United States alone. Fortunately, the field of maternal mental health has been growing, especially in the last few years, as clinicians and researchers are becoming increasingly aware of the need for information and treatment for those suffering.

The various terms used by the public (and with some practitioners as well) can be confusing, so I'll clarify them here. The "Baby Blues" are sometimes incorrectly called "mild postpartum depression." This is not the case. The Baby Blues are normal. Most mothers experience a few days of weepiness and feeling stressed, beginning the first week following delivery. Although they are not pleasant, the Baby Blues are relatively mild and should be gone by about two weeks postpartum. If the Baby Blues continue past the two week mark, then the condition becomes postpartum depression—even if the symptoms continue to be mild. Now the woman needs professional intervention instead of just sound support. Another note—postpartum mood and anxiety disorders can begin immediately after delivery and overlap the first two weeks (the Baby Blues period). If the symptoms are getting in the way of the woman's functioning and she has lost her perspective, is unable to sleep, has lost her appetite, is extremely anxious, or is acting strangely, she should find help immediately and not try to "wait it out." To illustrate, postpartum psychosis typically rears its head within the first two or three days postpartum.

It can also be confusing when all six of the postpartum mood and anxiety disorders are mistakenly lumped together under "postpartum depression." Postpartum depression is one of six disorders falling under the umbrella called "postpartum mood and anxiety disorders."

Postpartum Depression affects about 15 percent of new mothers and may begin any time during the first year postpartum. Symptoms include anxiety, lack of energy, forgetfulness, frequent crying, sleeping problems, low self-esteem, hopelessness, feeling overwhelmed, appetite problems, and irritability or anger.

Postpartum Bipolar Disorder is characterized by severe mood swings from an extremely elevated mood to severe depression. The elevated mood is called mania. In a manic episode, among other feelings, the woman may experience a decreased need for sleep, increased sex drive, inappropriately extreme happiness, speeding thoughts, impulsiveness, and an inflated ego.

Postpartum Panic Disorder involves heart palpitations, numbness and tingling, dizziness, hot or cold flashes, shaking, a fear of losing control, and claustrophobia.

Postpartum Posttraumatic Stress Disorder affects the woman with extreme anxiety, flashbacks to the trauma, and recurrent nightmares.

Postpartum Obsessive-Compulsive Disorder and **Postpartum Psychosis** will be discussed in detail later in this chapter.

TERMINOLOGY

The uniqueness of the postpartum disorders has not been outlined well in the DSM,[1] the *Diagnostic and Statistical Manual* used as a guide by clinicians. When the first DSM came out in 1952, the term "postpartum" was excluded entirely. Although the term postpartum is back in the official vocabulary, there is still no actual postpartum diagnosis. For example, although postpartum depression is informally referred to as a diagnosis, it is not one of the official diagnostic categories in the DSM. The clinician needs to add what's known as an "onset specifier" to the diagnosis, which states that the disorder began postpartum. So, it's implied, that the mood disorder is the same as if it occurs at any other time in one's life; the only part that's different is when it begins.

Both clinicians and clients have been confused by the official terminology for postpartum mood disorders. The Postpartum Onset Specifier blends all of the postpartum mood disorders into one. The Postpartum Onset Specifier states that the illness "with postpartum onset (can be applied to the current or most recent Major Depressive, Manic, or Mixed Episode in Major Depressive Disorder, Bipolar 1 Disorder, or Bipolar 11 Disorder; or to Brief Psychotic Disorder). Onset of episode within four weeks postpartum. In general, the symptomatology of the postpartum Major Depressive, Manic or Mixed Episode does not differ from the symptomatology in nonpostpartum mood episodes and may include psychotic features."[2] There is misinformation in this ambiguous description regarding time of onset and symptoms. Specialists in the field agree that this description is too restrictive—postpartum depression, for instance, may begin any time during the first postpartum. Also, the symptoms of all six disorders are combined to appear as if they belong to the same disorder. Important as well, according to the DSM, the postpartum mood disorders are not considered to warrant their own diagnoses.

Present terminology confuses not only those responsible for medical care, but also the criminal justice system. The result is often to sacrifice the rights of women suffering. A woman, for instance, who has postpartum obsessive-compulsive disorder (OCD), might be reported to Child Protective Services if she admits to having thoughts of harming her infant. This agency may turn her in to the police if her symptoms are not recognized properly as harmless to her baby. Her baby may then be placed in protective custody or foster care. In addition, women with postpartum psychosis who commit infanticide often find themselves in prison rather than in a hospital receiving the medical attention they desperately need.

WHEN CLINICIANS MAKE MISTAKES

Misdiagnoses can cause a lot of difficulty. For instance, if a woman with bipolar disorder—a condition that is characterized by extreme mood swings—is depressed at the time of her evaluation, and the practitioner doesn't ask her the right questions, she can easily be diagnosed as having postpartum depression. The concern is that this woman may be given an antidepressant, and an antidepressant by itself can throw the woman into a manic episode. The two particular postpartum disorders about which there seems to be the most confusion are postpartum obsessive-compulsive disorder (OCD) and postpartum psychosis (PPP). They are often mistaken for one another, and this can cause serious undue trauma for all concerned. I will describe them in greater detail now, to help differentiate these two distinct disorders.

Postpartum OCD

What complicates matters greatly is that moms who have postpartum OCD are very much afraid that they have PPP. Postpartum OCD may show up in a number of ways, and not all of the symptoms are experienced by every mother with OCD. The particular symptom that seems to disturb these moms the most—and causes much confusion for practitioners—is scary thoughts of the baby being harmed. Sometimes these thoughts involve the mother herself doing the harming. Mothers with OCD are terrified of their thoughts, and ashamed, especially before they understand that the thoughts have nothing to do with their character or ability to mother. Due to the scary nature of these thoughts, they don't trust themselves. They are thinking, "If I'm capable of thinking these horrible things, then what will stop me from doing them?" If she's envisioning herself dropping her baby over a balcony, she's anxious that she'll actually follow through and do it. There's not one case on record of a woman, due to postpartum OCD, ever following through on one of her thoughts. She's just afraid that she will. If anything, these moms are overprotective. Scary thoughts of the baby being harmed by her or someone else can vary tremendously in content, but there are some that are especially common. A fear of dropping or throwing the baby from a high place and cutting or stabbing the baby with a sharp object are two of the most frequently reported thoughts. Any common innocuous household object can suddenly trigger a scary obsession. As already stated, these women are the most protective mothers on the planet. They're the ones who can anticipate potential danger, and their protective instinct has gone a bit over the line. For instance, they can walk into a room and immediately pick out every thing that might be hazardous to the baby—a sharp edge of a coffee table, an unlocked baby gate, and so on. They may also find danger where there isn't any realistically. Rationally they know their fears are far-fetched, but it doesn't stop their minds from chattering and envisioning the worst. They are obsessing about the worst possible event that may happen to their child—that the child may get hurt or killed. And the most terrifying thing that her anxious mind can find to obsess about is that she may be the person who does the harming. A mom with OCD (or any other postpartum mood disorder) does not want to hurt her child—she has the exact opposite intention. Her worst fear is not being able to keep her baby safe, even from herself.

Professionals who haven't received specialized training in postpartum OCD sometimes wrongly assume the woman has postpartum psychosis. This often causes undue trauma and suffering for all concerned. This particular misdiagnosis is especially damaging to the mother, since she is already worrying that she may be psychotic or will snap and become psychotic. She fears that, worst of all, if she is psychotic she'll lose control and become a danger to her baby. With this misdiagnosis, her fears are confirmed and often, sadly, by the people who are supposed to be helping her—her healthcare professionals.

Sometimes these healthcare professionals hospitalize the mother or have her baby taken away, which further convinces her that she's a danger to her child. This unnecessary damage and trauma, which unfortunately is still happening, can take quite a while to undo. When a scary piece of news is released about a mom killing her baby (as in the case of Andrea Yates), the moms with postpartum OCD are worried that they'll become like the mother in the news. We in the field are flooded with calls from moms with OCD whenever there's a news report of this kind. And they need quite a bit of reassuring. The fact that their thoughts and behaviors are distressing to them is a good sign. Their feelings about their thoughts are one way we can tell the difference between OCD and PPP. (If a mom is psychotic, chances are she would not be calling a medical care provider for help for herself. There are exceptions to that, but usually this is the case.) Mothers with OCD are calling because they know there's something wrong with their thinking. They're aware of not being normal and about having thoughts they would not normally have. They can tell they're off balance because they are in this reality.

It's also important to reassure them that OCD does not turn into psychosis. The two conditions are quite different. Moms who are suffering only from OCD are not a danger to their babies. Moms with OCD will go to great lengths to protect their children—even from themselves. These moms may go in another room and leave the baby safe in the crib for a little while as a precaution since they don't trust themselves. A mother with OCD dreads being left alone with her child. She's highly anxious and overwhelmed.

The greatest risk in this situation is that moms with OCD may so intensely (and mistakenly) fear that they are a danger to their children that they may commit suicide in an effort to protect them. They will do away with themselves before they'd ever hurt their children.

Sometimes this mom's anxiety leads to superstitious thinking. If, for instance, the mom with OCD has an obsession about her baby dying, she might convince herself that if she doesn't continually check the child's breathing, or doesn't fix the baby's blanket in that exact way a certain number of times, something terrible might happen—the baby might die by smothering or stopping breathing. And then the mom may go off into a scenario in her mind that her baby's death will be all her fault. She may even imagine going to prison. She can envision all of this very vividly like she's watching snippets of horror movies replaying over and over in her head. Often the fear is that something negative will happen if the behavior (like checking the blanket or baby's breathing) is not indulged. Safety is always the theme. She's having these obsessive thoughts and also indulging in compulsive behaviors in an attempt to keep her child safe.

Excerpt from **Postpartum Depression for Dummies***: Symptoms of* **OCD**

- *A need to count things repetitively, such as bottles*
- *A need to check things repetitively, such as doors to ensure that they're locked, and the baby's breathing*
- *A need to constantly clean and tidy up*
- *Germ phobia*
- *A need to have things "just so"*
- *Terrifying images or thoughts of harming the baby or watching the baby be harmed*
- *Intense shame and disgust about these thoughts*
- *Behaving in ways that reduce the anxiety about the thoughts they're having (for example, hiding sharp objects)*
- *Distrust of herself, especially when alone with her baby*

Postpartum Psychosis (PPP)

PPP is very different from OCD. A mom with PPP may be operating in two realities simultaneously. She understands what is expected of her and what is considered normal to the rest of the world, and she has her own reality occurring at the same time. Her reality dictates what she determines needs to be done and how she perceives events around her, whether or not anyone else believes her. This mom often floats in and out of normal reality. It's impossible to count on her being rational from one moment to the next. She may be completely rational one moment, and the next moment she may be in a psychotic state. One minute she'll be talking to herself or others and not making sense (delusional, strange statements) and the next she'll be able to carry on a normal conversation.

Excerpt from **Postpartum Depression for Dummies***: Symptoms of* **PPP** *(additions to the excerpt are not in italics)*

- *Auditory hallucinations (hearing things others don't)*: Sometimes these can be general sounds like laughter or talking or "special *messages*" she perceives as being meant only for her coming *from the TV, radio, computer, or newspaper*. Or, they may be commands telling her to do something, including instructing her to harm her baby.
- *Bizarre thoughts* including those *about needing to kill her baby*
- *Confusion*
- *Disorientation*
- *Extreme agitation*

- *Insomnia (difficulty sleeping)*
- *Paranoia (false beliefs that others are trying to harm her or her children)*: Often this is directed at those closest to her, her partner, family, and/or doctors. She may lie, become hostile, angry, or obstinate, even regarding insignificant topics.
- Hallucinations: these may include *tactile hallucinations (feeling things that aren't there, for instance spiders crawling up her arm), visual hallucinations (seeing things others don't)*, olfactory (smelling things others don't), or even tasting things others don't.
- She may feel like some outside force is taking her over and controlling her actions.
- Loss of focus (such as not being able to follow a plot)
- Loss of cognitive ability (unable to answer questions of "why" or do mathematical problems)
- Loss of ability to read
- Delusions (false beliefs firmly held): Many of these have common themes, such as religion or persecution.

It is not necessary or usual for a woman with postpartum psychosis to exhibit all of these symptoms. And, the symptoms may come and go. For example, a woman may be able to read at one point in the day but then lose the ability later.

Note—many normal new moms report hearing their babies cry when their babies are not actually crying. This is a common and normal phenomenon. If this occurs by itself without the other symptoms listed, it does not indicate a problem.

THE UNIVERSAL MESSAGE

You're not alone. One to three women per thousand become psychotic after delivering a baby.

You're not to blame. The experts are in agreement that there are biochemical components to this disorder. The brain chemistry changes in a number of ways, many of which we aren't sure of yet. This disorder (as in the case of all the postpartum disorders listed) has nothing to do with a character deficiency.

You will be well. This is a very treatable disorder, as all of the postpartum disorders are. It is considered to be an acute episode, not chronic, when proper help is received.

PPP comes with a 5% suicide rate and a 4% infanticide rate. Psychotic mothers do not want to kill their babies, but they may feel a need to do so. Andrea Yates did not want to kill her children—she loved them very much. In her delusional state, she felt there was a need to, in order to protect them. That is a huge difference. A mother's paranoia may make her believe that neighbors are out to get her or her children. Sometimes these mothers experience an inability to read. They literally cannot decipher the printed page—the words may as well be hieroglyphics. If she can read, she still may have difficulty processing the meaning of what she read. She may not be able to follow a plot of a movie or TV show. Another common symptom is a sudden religious preoccupation—an obsession with religion or religious figures. This can happen even if she isn't religious at all in her normal life. She may obsess about Jesus, Satan, or both. A mom with postpartum psychosis may also be deceitful. She knows what the rest of the world believes, and may say or do anything that she feels she must do, including lie. In her delusional mind, she may think she has to do certain things in order to protect herself or the child(ren), and she may lie in the process. Most likely she is not normally a deceitful person. But, in her psychotic state, if she feels threatened or is trying to protect her babies, she'll do or say whatever is necessary. This mother almost always admits to what she has done if she commits infanticide. She is often the one to call 911 and report on herself, "I killed my baby." But she is not always honest as to what happened. She may know the rest of the world is not thinking the way she is, so she hides the illness from others. Sometimes she is honest, and she recounts every step and the delusional reasons why she felt she had to take those steps. But at other times, she may concoct some story or hide the body. That does not mean that she was sane at the time of the event.

Postpartum psychosis typically begins during the first few days following the delivery. If the brain chemistry is going to cause PPP, it usually does so pretty quickly after the baby is born, so it overlaps the Baby Blues period. More than half of PPP cases begin the first week and more than 75 percent begin before the first two weeks.

Postpartum psychosis is always considered to be a medical emergency—one should never wait it out to see if it goes away by itself. This is much too risky for both the mother and the child(ren).

RARELY DOES A MOM IN A PSYCHOTIC STATE REACH OUT FOR HELP

This may be due to her paranoia and not trusting the rest of the world, but often she isn't reaching out because she doesn't recognize that anything is wrong with her. It is usually a family member, a partner, a friend, or the doctor who contacts a therapist after the woman has been hospitalized or when they feel she's acting odd, and they want her to receive an assessment. These moms are usually too ill to find help on their own, and waiting for them to initiate can lead to tragedy. This is even more reason for those around new mothers to be observant.

On the other hand, just because a new mother is aware something's wrong and does ask for help, she should not automatically be dismissed as not having PPP. She needs screening for this disorder like any other new mother. As a matter of fact, many of these mothers have a strong feeling that something is very wrong—either with themselves, their children, their partners, and so on. They may call a doctor or therapist during one of their more rational moments. The times when I've been contacted directly by a mother with PPP, there has been a variety of emotions expressed by them—mainly fear about hallucinations, or sounding dazed, confused, and inarticulate. As a practitioner, I immediately try to get another adult on the phone who is close to her. Without being alarmist, I calmly but strongly suggest that he or she takes the new mom to the nearest hospital for an evaluation. I let the support person know that the mom may have postpartum psychosis and she needs help immediately. I also make sure the support person understands the gravity of the situation and inform him or her that the mom should not be left alone or alone with the baby even for an instant until it's known what's going on with her.

There are many myths about postpartum psychosis. One is that postpartum psychosis is always apparent to those around the woman. In truth, it may be difficult to spot, depending on her symptoms. Although sometimes the condition may be obvious, many of these women are able to present themselves as normal to the outside world. They may be dressed as usual and able to participate in their regular daily activities. If she does not share what's going on in her delusional mind, and she's acting normally, it may be difficult to pick up unless you are around her a lot. That's why close family members and friends are in the best position to notice something awry and get her help. OBs are also in an advantageous spot to identify psychosis (or other postpartum disorders) if they screen their postpartum patients (as all OB offices should do) for mental health disorders. There are a number of excellent screening tools used to detect postpartum depression such as the Postpartum Depression Screening Scale and the Edinburgh Postnatal Depression Scale. However, none of these tools are specifically used for postpartum psychosis. If a mother is high risk for PPP, hopefully this information is in her file, and the OB will be watching for signs and asking the appropriate questions to determine her mental health.

Another myth is that once a woman has had a postpartum psychosis, she will always have mental illness. If she has schizophrenia, she may always be challenged with mental illness. But if she was hit with a postpartum psychosis and doesn't have a history of a chronic psychotic disorder, she has every reason to believe that once it's gone, it's gone. Even if she had a mental illness (like schizophrenia) before she delivered her baby, the acute postpartum episode will end, as long as she receives proper help. All of the postpartum disorders are considered to be acute (temporary)—not chronic (ongoing).

PPP RISK AND TREATMENT

If a woman has bipolar disorder or has experienced a psychotic episode in the past, she is high risk for postpartum psychosis. If she has a family history of either bipolar disorder or psychosis (such as schizophrenia), she has between a 20 and 50 percent chance of experiencing PPP. And if she's had a previous psychosis postpartum, her risk jumps up to 75 percent. But this illness also strikes women with no history of mental disorder. "Postpartum women with milder forms of mood-swing disorders (such as bipolar II) are probably the most underdiagnosed and mistreated group," researchers and authors Sichel and Driscoll report. "Their rapidly disintegrating mental health comes as a complete surprise, not only to them and their families but also to their health-care providers."[3]

However, some researchers believe even in these women a careful, detailed history can identify those at risk. According to Sichel and Driscoll, "Indeed, we have come to believe that it is *rare* to find no evidence of previous mood shifts in women who experience an initial episode of psychosis postpartum. *The key is in taking a careful and sensitive history, so that any past disturbances may be identified.*"[4]

In fact, when Sichel and Driscoll studied the charts of the first thirty women to be admitted to a psychiatric mother-baby unit, they found that twenty-six of them had diagnosable mood issues before pregnancy but had just lived with them and not sought help. These symptoms that were present before pregnancy put these women into a high risk category, but they did not know it because careful histories were not taken. "They could have been diagnosed quite easily during their pregnancies if someone had asked the right questions. And once they delivered their babies, a preventative treatment plan could have been instituted and the severity of the illness curtailed, avoiding hospitalization and distress to the mothers and their families."[5] Too often this is not done and chances for prevention are lost. Then the best she can hope for is a knowledgeable practitioner and effective treatment of the psychosis.

Psychosis is very treatable, but the mother needs to be in a hospital. If for any reason she cannot be hospitalized, a responsible adult needs to watch her every second, including in the bathroom. One never knows what might go through her head at any given moment, so she should never be left alone or alone with the baby until she's more stable. After the postpartum psychosis is treated, often there's a depression underlying it that needs treatment as well.

OCD AND PPP TOGETHER

It would be easy if postpartum women could simply fit neatly into one of these six postpartum disorder categories. These disorders are separated, mainly for the purposes of research and treatment, but women don't fit neatly into these groups—there can be combinations. So a woman, for example, may have postpartum depression or postpartum OCD along with a panic disorder. Or she may experience OCD with depression, PTSD with OCD, or either of these with panic and depression. Here's where it can get tricky. OCD and PPP are completely different disorders. But, it's possible that both of these disorders may emerge concurrently. This is probably the toughest combination to handle, both for the clinicians and for the moms. Chances are the mom with OCD does not have psychosis; however, she needs a thorough assessment to make sure. Almost always the practitioner will be able to give her reassurance that she has OCD and she's not a danger to her baby.

A qualified practitioner—a professional who understands the difference between these two disorders—should screen the woman carefully. This professional needs to be able to distinguish between a scary thought or fear of not being able to trust herself, and a psychotic person who has the intent to harm (in order to protect) her baby.

If a medical doctor suspects that one of his or her patients may be dealing with a postpartum mood or anxiety disorder, a referral should be made to a psychotherapist who has received specialized training in this field. Postpartum Support International is the leading organization offering this training. You can visit Postpartum.net for more information on the yearly conference, pre-conference training for professionals, and other recommended conferences being held around the world.

As research in the field progresses, more practitioners are trained to screen new moms and provide assessments, so an increasing number of mothers and their families are receiving help quickly. Hopefully soon, the terminology in the DSM will recognize these disorders as distinct, and they will have diagnoses all their own as they deserve. This advancement will make not only the diagnosis clearer, but it should also lead to quicker and more appropriate treatment. With excellent books spreading the word, such as the one you're reading now, those who are suffering, along with their loved ones, are gathering needed information about prevention and treatment options.

Chapter 2

Psychological Views and Treatment

Shoshana Bennett, PhD

As far back as women have been having babies, it is believed that a certain percentage of them suffered from postpartum psychiatric illness. Postpartum psychosis (PPP) was first formally recognized as a disorder in the mid-1800s. Research has indicated that the percentage of women who are affected today has not changed since then.

Postpartum psychosis is rare (one to three women per thousand), and is always considered to be a medical emergency. Although PPP can occur after any birth, it is most often experienced after the first. Once a mom has experienced PPP, she's high risk for another episode after she gives birth again. The risk of recurrence will be discussed at the end of this chapter. This mom needs to be hospitalized immediately for treatment, in order to keep her and her family safe.

Without proper treatment, there is a 5 percent suicide rate and a 4 percent infanticide rate. One of the biggest challenges associated with providing treatment for women with PPP is that these women often resist treatment. This reluctance (or downright refusal) of care is due to the symptoms of the illness itself. The woman with PPP may be distrusting or paranoid of anyone who tries to help her. Or, in her delusional condition, she does not believe that there's anything wrong with her. Sometimes she physically fights in a rage when a loved one tries to bring her in to the hospital. State laws vary within the United States regarding how to handle the situation that arises when a woman refuses treatment.

CAUSES

Researchers do not know for sure what causes PPP, but it's generally accepted that biochemical changes in the brain during pregnancy

and after delivery are involved. There are other factors that may contribute to the woman's risk. Some of these factors include a personal or
family history of mental illness (especially bipolar disorder or schizophrenia), past trauma, stress, depleted nutrition, thyroid dysfunction,
and sleep deprivation.

MORE ON SYMPTOMS

Many of the most common symptoms associated with PPP are listed
and discussed in chapter one. You may notice that the content of the
woman's conversation may reflect her disjointed thoughts; she may be
saying very odd things that make no sense.

Her behavior may also be odd, bizarre, and unusual as compared to
her normal self. When a woman with PPP is set in her false beliefs
(delusions), it will not help or be effective if you try to convince her
otherwise. Actually, that can backfire and make her more entrenched
in the delusion. If you try to reason with her, she may spend lots of
energy trying to convince you that she's right, and that in turn
strengthens her false beliefs.

Difficulty sleeping is usually present. It's a warning sign for any of
the postpartum mood or anxiety disorders, but with psychosis the
insomnia can be severe. Any new mom who cannot sleep at night
when the baby is sleeping for a few nights in a row needs help (it
doesn't mean that the mom is psychotic necessarily, but she needs
some kind of treatment right away).

MEDICATION

As with treating any psychotic episode, most doctors agree that
other physiological causes need to be ruled out. A thorough physical
exam and blood tests are frequently ordered, so that the doctor can
assess whether there's an organic medical illness causing the psychosis.
These may include thyroid disease, seizure disorders, drugs, infection,
or renal disease. A CAT scan may also be prescribed in order to be
sure a brain tumor or other abnormal mass is not present.

Medications to treat the PPP are almost always prescribed to allevi-
ate the symptoms. As with any other serious disorder, prognosis is best
the sooner treatment is begun. Early intervention is key. The longer the
woman is left untreated, the less effective a medication might be. Plus,
the more dangerous and damaging it will be for her and her entire
family. Among others, commonly prescribed antipsychotic medications
used to treat PPP are Haldol, Risperidal, Zyprexa, and Clozaril. Most.
women are treated with a pill form of medication, but some who are
not able or not willing to swallow medication may be given injections
of medication. Two of these medications commonly administered are

Risperidone and Olanzapine. As with all medications, antipsychotic medications pass into the mother's breast milk. Consequently, if the mom wishes to continue to breastfeed, often the baby is monitored for extra drowsiness. You can check with motherrisk.org for more information on safety with medications while breastfeeding.

Until she is mentally stable, someone needs to be present with the mother, never leaving her alone or alone with her baby, even when she's breastfeeding. This is necessary to ensure the safety of the mother and baby. If she cannot be admitted to an inpatient facility, which is strongly suggested, a responsible adult needs to be on duty with her at all times until she stabilizes. It's ideal if the mother can remain in close contact with her baby and other children as she's treated, so those relationships can be nurtured. Mother-baby units are few and far between, but if that arrangement is available, it's excellent as long as it's appropriate for the needs of the family. But, until she's recovered sufficiently and is "herself" and rational steadily for a few weeks, it is not safe to leave her alone or alone with her child(ren) without careful supervision. Occasionally, due to the specific symptoms of the mother (such as explosive anger), it will be better for her and her children not to bring them together for visits until she's more normal.

Antipsychotic medication may only be needed short-term in many cases. The response to mood stabilizers and antipsychotic medications is usually quick. As mentioned in chapter one, typically after the psychotic symptoms are alleviated, an underlying depression needs treatment before the mom becomes completely well. Once the psychosis lifts, individual counseling, group counseling or support groups, and couples counseling can be of great benefit. She may have been traumatized during her psychotic episode or during her treatment. In any case, she'll be scared about what happened to her, and most likely fearful that it could happen again. Postpartum depression support groups can often be quite helpful, but the mom who has been psychotic may feel alienated from the rest of the group, since the other moms didn't actually "lose their mind" and may not be able to relate. The group facilitator may need to work extra hard to help the mom feel included. If her OB, group facilitator, or other practitioner can connect her directly with another survivor of PPP, these women can form their own type of support group.

The process of full physical and psychological recovery may take a while. The entire family needs support and education. Close family members—especially partners—need educating and counseling, since they may have experienced their own trauma during this process. No matter what, they will need their own help and support of various kinds as they are providing the necessary care to the recovering woman. They also need to know what to watch for in case of a relapse or future psychotic episode. The child(ren) may need emotional help, either alone or with their mom to ensure their relationships are secure and healthy.

Careful monitoring and follow-up is important. If the couple plans on having more children, family planning and medical consultation should happen as soon as possible. The couple should not wait until pregnancy for a number of reasons. First, the couple should receive information about how to space the births of their children. Having babies too close together is riskier for relapse. Also, the mom may be taking a medication that is not recommended for pregnancy, so weaning off or changing medications might be indicated.

Every expecting couple—not only those at high risk for PPP—should have a plan of action in place before the baby comes. But in the case of those at high risk for PPP, this plan is crucial. If the woman is on medication during pregnancy, ideally a psychiatrist (or another MD, if necessary) is monitoring her moods to make sure she's on the correct dosage. In addition, this mom needs excellent sleep when the baby comes, since sleep deprivation renders her even more vulnerable to a psychotic episode. Specific nutrients should be in her daily diet, some in supplement form, and she needs physical and emotional support. It is always wise to increase the frequency of therapy sessions before delivery and for about three months following the birth.

ELECTROCONVULSIVE THERAPY (ECT)

I haven't met a woman who looks forward to ECT, but many have expressed gratitude for its availability. These moms understand that without ECT, they might have ended up like Andrea Yates. Andrea Yates, who took the lives of her children in the midst of a psychotic episode postpartum, was offered this treatment before that terrible event occurred. Possibly due to her fear, confusion, distrust, and misunderstanding of ECT, she refused the treatment. Although there's no way to say for sure, ECT may have saved her and her family from the tragedy that followed.

This therapy involves sending a tiny bit of electricity to the brain. There are chemical changes triggered by the electricity that can reduce the symptoms of PPP. ECT is usually well tolerated and works rapidly. It's typically used to treat severe postpartum depression and psychosis. This is a humane treatment—not scary or painful. The woman is given a short-acting general anesthetic along with a muscle relaxant. ECT is often administered in a course of a few sessions (often six to eight), depending upon how many she needs. Immediately following a session, she may have a headache or feel nauseous. There is typically memory loss, usually temporary short-term memory. ECT has about an 80 percent success rate. Many countries don't understand why the United States is so slow to offer a suffering woman ECT, and why it's usually considered the last resort. These countries wonder why a woman may be put through trials of many medications and be suffering for a long time before the treatment is suggested. With psychosis, ECT can be the quickest and best option to take, considering the severity of the disorder and depending upon the individual woman's response to medication.

When medication hasn't been effective for the mom, after ECT she often finds that the medication works—the ECT works for the brain like re-booting a computer. ECT can also be used effectively in combination with medication, so it needn't be considered an either/or decision. Breastfeeding can continue for moms going through ECT treatments.

COMPLEMENTARY HEALING METHODS

As already discussed, medication (and usually hospitalization) will be needed to treat PPP. In addition, there are other treatment methods that can be used concurrently with medicine. These methods can help heal the underlying causes of the psychotic episode. Addressing specific nutritional, emotional, and environmental needs can help prevent another episode.

Alternative health practitioners working with these moms use a variety of tests (saliva, blood, urine, or hair samples, typically). These professionals, including nutritionists, chiropractors, and acupuncturists, test the women for imbalances. Among other common findings, they frequently report that the women have mineral deficiencies, thyroid dysfunction, and an elevated level of copper. There are foods; vitamins and minerals, such as B6, iron, magnesium, antioxidants, and omega-3 fatty acids; and other particular substances that can help restore the necessary balance in chemistry and affect the neurotransmitters (brain chemistry) in a positive way. There is also evidence to suggest that when certain nutrients are present (such as folate or folic acid), medications may work better, even if they hadn't worked previously. *A Natural Guide to Pregnancy and Postpartum Health* (Raffelock) goes into great detail about these nutrients.

Sleep deprivation is a very important factor that always needs addressing in the case of PPP. Chronic sleep deprivation affects brain chemistry negatively, and can make a psychosis worse. Many professionals in the field feel that sleep deprivation can even cause the psychosis, but all are in agreement that it's certainly a prevalent symptom. If a new mother is not able to sleep at all at night when her baby is sleeping, she needs help immediately. Especially when a woman reports not being able to sleep for a few days (and nights) in a row, this is a warning sign. In addition to immediate help, she will need a longer plan of action to ensure solid, uninterrupted sleep at night in order to fully recover. A natural sleep aid, "sleep glasses," are worn two or three hours before bed. The glasses help the natural melatonin in the brain start flowing. There are already studies showing significant improvement in people with bipolar illness who use this method. Check ClearSky-Inc.com for more information.

Other modalities such as homeopathy and acupuncture have been reported as well to help patients recover. More research is needed before these methods can be established in the standard medical litera- ture. If you choose to use these methods, make sure you're working with a knowledgeable practitioner and your doctor is aware of what you're doing. For instance, there are herbs that may be prescribed to you that should not be mixed with certain medications that you're tak- ing. The Center for Complementary and Alternative Medicine has a good Web site for more information on these methods and others, at http://nccam.nih.gov.

When the mom is still in a psychotic state, it may be difficult to make exercise part of her regimen, but once she's feeling more normal, it can help her with the rest of her recovery. If she is manic and able to work off some of her extra energy with exercise, it probably won't hurt her, but it won't "cure" her. She will need other modes of treatment in addition to exercise.

RISK OF RECURRENCE AND PREVENTION

Women who receive appropriate treatment are expected to com- pletely recover. The recovered mom may not ever experience another psychotic episode again. However, she and her loved ones need to understand that her risk of having a PPP in the future after another baby is 50 percent greater than women who haven't had it. There is some evidence that her risk decreases if she spreads out the time pe- riod between pregnancies. There are prevention techniques, both medi- cal and non-medical, used to help ward off a subsequent PPP. It's crucial that a high risk mother receives medical advice well before the baby is born. Whenever possible, the woman or couple should meet with a practitioner who has the appropriate clinical expertise regarding psychiatric medication in pregnancy and postpartum. Ideally, this med- ical planning should happen before she gets pregnant, in case medica- tions need to be weaned off or switched before pregnancy. During pregnancy she needs careful monitoring for mood changes. Some women who have experienced PPP decide not to have more children. Those who have another child often decide, with their doctors' guid- ance, to start taking medication immediately upon delivery. They don't want to wait and see if another psychosis begins—it was so scary for them last time, they want to do all they can in advance to help prevent it.

Prescribing lithium carbonate to the mother after delivery as a pre- vention technique is controversial, but it has been shown to be quite effective. The connection between PPP and bipolar disorder is well established, hence the use of prescribing lithium, a mood stabilizer often used in the treatment of bipolar disorder. Mood stabilizers, as the name suggests, help balance mood swings. Lithium is not safe when breastfeeding. So, the plan of which medications will be used needs to be discussed, taking into consideration what works for the woman and also her wish to breastfeed. Depakote, another mood stabilizer, is approved for use while breastfeeding.

CONCLUSION

Postpartum psychosis is very treatable, and there are ways to minimize its occurrence and severity. With pre-pregnancy planning, monitoring during pregnancy by her family and team of professionals, plus an excellent plan of action following the birth, even a high risk mom can emerge from the pregnancy and birth both healthy and happy.

Chapter 3

Postpartum Psychosis Across History and in the Media Today

WHY DIDN'T I KNOW?

In 1998, I faithfully attended childbirth classes, went to a Lamaze meeting, and took a special natural-childbirth class. I read *Parents* and *Baby Talk* magazines. I compulsively read books on childbirth, including the popular *What to Expect When You're Expecting*. I did research on vaccinations. I thought I was prepared and well informed. I was wrong. Nothing I was told or read prepared me for my actual childbirth and postpartum experience.

It was not until the early days of the twenty-first century that I learned the name of the illness that devastated me after the birth of my first baby two years earlier: postpartum psychosis. While on bedrest expecting twins, I began to search for information on postpartum psychosis (PPP). I Googled it but got no hits. I searched in all my baby books. I found nothing except the occasional reference describing it as "rare" and "dangerous." None of the books described symptoms, frequency, risk factors, treatments, or the like.

I thought I simply had limited resources and would find more complete information when I was able to go to a library or a bookstore. Even there, however, I found little of substance. At one university library I found a practitioner's resource book that listed PPP. Unfortunately, instead of bothering to list symptoms, it stated that doing so was unnecessary as it would be obvious to anyone around the woman that she was psychotic. Well, I knew that was wrong. If it was obvious, I would have been diagnosed—but I wasn't. I kept searching.

There *were* books with valuable information on PPP. James Hamilton's *A Picture Puzzle* was published in 1992 (now out of print). Carol Dix's wonderful book *The New Mother Syndrome*, published in 1985, was probably already out of print by the year 2000. There were also many professional articles. But there was woefully little *available* to someone like me.

My oldest child is now ten years old. And things have changed. It seems everyone is familiar with the term PPP, generally in association with the Yates tragedy. There are more books that mention it and even offer details. On a recent trip to a bookstore I discovered that many of the general books on childbirth and new motherhood mentioned PPP and listed some of the symptoms.

I Googled "postpartum psychosis" again in July of 2008, and I got about 11,000 hits. It seems the tide has turned. But the more things change, the more they stay the same. On one recent trip to a big-box bookstore, the shelves on pregnancy and motherhood had no books on postpartum depression. When I asked the kind, slightly bookish-looking young woman at the information kiosk to do a search for "postpartum depression," it led to a few books in the psychology section and one in self-help. I then asked her to search for "postpartum psychosis." They had only one book, *Breaking Point* by Suzy Spencer, in the "True Crime" section. I asked why there were no books on postpartum mood disorders (PPMDs) in the large portion of shelves devoted to pregnant and new mothers. She remarked that new moms probably "don't want to see books like that." Another bookstore had one book on PPMDs on its approximately 15 x 7 feet of shelving for books on pregnancy and parenting—Shoshana Bennett's *Postpartum Depression for Dummies*.

And yet doctors tell me that their patients don't want to hear about "stuff like that."

And—a new mother, crying so hard she is gasping, asks me, "Why didn't anyone tell me?"

Indeed, why is it taking so long for us to wake up to this deadly but treatable condition that every year causes so much heartache and preventable tragedies?

POSTPARTUM PSYCHOSIS IS NOT NEW—IT WAS JUST LOST

Postpartum psychosis has gone by a number of names.[1] Hippocrates described postpartum psychiatric illness in the fourth century BC.[2] But the first systematic study of mental illness related to childbearing was reported by Jean Etienne Dominique Esquirol in 1838.[3] In the mid-1800s Louis Victor Marcé continued this work.[4] Experts in the nineteenth century studied and wrote papers on the unique features of postpartum psychiatric illness. In fact, Hilary Marland in the book *Dangerous Motherhood, Insanity and Childbirth in Victorian Britain* states, "[B]y the mid-nineteenth century no textbook on the diseases of women would be complete without a section on puerperal insanity."[5] But in the twentieth century, "[I]nterest in postpartum emotional disorders lapsed in the U.S. after the American Psychiatric Association removed the concept from the first *Diagnostic and Statistical Manual of Mental Disorders (DSM)...."*[6] PPMDs were not omitted from the *DSM* because women did not experience mood disorders postpartum but rather because those disorders were not considered sufficient to constitute their own category.

A brief summary of how this came to be:[7] First, because the specific causes of mental illness were and are largely unknown, the identifications are based on clusters of symptoms—these fall into three broad categories: disorders in thinking (schizoform); disorders of emotional reactions, or "affective" disorders (bipolar); and those where toxic agents or trauma interfere with the functions of the nervous system (toxic-exhaustive psychoses or organic psychoses). Most varieties of mental illness could fit into one of these, with one outstanding exception—psychiatric illness after childbirth. PPP patients might cycle or shift from symptoms typical of one to those of another or even exhibit symptoms of all three categories at the same time. They might exhibit mood changes such as depression or mania (bipolar), along with delirium and confusion (organic psychosis) and delusions (schizoform). "Some ... suggested that these undisciplined patients be tagged according to the symptom pattern which was most prominent at the time of the diagnosis."[8] The official line on this is that psychiatric illnesses after childbearing are not significantly different from those that occur in the general population. We know postpartum psychosis tends to come on extremely rapidly, but other psychoses may sometimes come on rapidly as well. And although mixed symptoms are typical in PPP, they may occur in non-postpartum people as well. PPP women have higher rates of delusions than non-postpartum psychotic women, but that does not mean non-postpartum women won't have delusions with psychosis. Finally, although typical and identifiable symptoms occur that keep PPP from fitting neatly into one of the existing three categories, it is not a fourth category—it does not contain symptoms not found in other illnesses—but it is rather an illness with a mix of symptoms from the existing three.

PPP may be diagnosed as "psychosis not otherwise specified" (a-typical psychosis) ... , "schizophreniform disorder ... and bipolar disorder, mixed...."[9] Lead researchers and authors note, "None of these named categories nor official descriptions convey any indication of the unique qualities and hazards of postpartum illness."[10]

Unfortunately, because these disorders are no longer considered distinct, "the more expectant approach, which saw puerperal insanity as a condition to be watched for and guarded against as it invaded the family home, [is] to a large extent lost."[11] This is evident in the missed diagnoses, inaccurate diagnoses, and failure to take preventative measures for those at risk.

Doctors' comments once indicated an understanding of the unique nature of the illness. These included the risk of harm ("Every precaution must be taken to prevent her doing injury to herself, to the infant, or her friends");[12] and the rapid and severe onset ("[A]cts of violence, sometimes suicide, are in this stage committed before the nature of the malady is suspected").[13] Sichel and Driscoll note, "The calamities we have described highlight the disconnections in our health system among obstetrics, gynecology, psychiatry, and pediatrics. Few clinicians realize how effectively appropriate intervention can avert tragedies."[14]

Although many historical accounts of barbaric treatment of the mentally ill exist, in the nineteenth century PPP women were often treated gently and with great care to avoid exacerbating their condition. Now, "the gentle, painstaking regimes of care were to a large extent lost, and puerperal insanity took on a darker and more menacing aspect."[15]

When public knowledge of this illness is limited to cases of infanticide it serves to perpetuate the stigma and ignorance women with this condition face. It also legitimizes the de-humanization and harsh treatment of those afflicted.

RECLAIMING AN IDENTITY: THE RISE OF A MOVEMENT

Without a distinct diagnosis, postpartum illness became "a condition without an identity."[16] But interest began to re-awaken among both professionals and laypersons, and in the 1980s the most prominent organizations that concern themselves with postpartum illness were formed.

In 1980, Ian Brockington called for an international conference of postpartum disorders in response to a postpartum tragedy. Out of this conference, Ian Brockington, James Hamilton, Ramesh "Channi" Kumar, and others launched the scientific arm of the postpartum movement, the Marcé Society, named after Dr. Louis Marcé. "The principal aim of the society is to promote, facilitate and communicate about research into all aspects of the mental health of women, their infants, and partners around the time of childbirth. This involves a broad range of research activities ranging from basic science through health services research."[17]

Around the same time that the Marcé society formed, grassroots organizations offering and encouraging social support also formed. In the United States, the best known of these were Depression After Delivery (D.A.D.) and Postpartum Support International (PSI). PSI has now absorbed D.A.D. to form one organization. The PSI Web site states, "Founded in 1987 to eliminate denial and ignorance of emotional health related to childbirth."[18] For almost 20 years PSI operated out of the home of founder Jane Honikman.

In 2001 another tragedy, the case of Andrea Yates, raised the profile and public awareness of this illness. Subsequently, PSI has experienced significant growth. This growth is evident in the PSI budget. The 1999–2000 PSI proposed budget listed revenues of $13,230. By 2002–2003 revenues were $101,400.[19]

In 1997, PSI had nineteen U.S. coordinators and three international contacts. In 2008, there were one hundred U.S. coordinators and forty international contacts. In addition, there are now special coordinators who handle topics including online, dads-partners, men with PPMDs, Spanish, military, and regional.[20]

This growth is particularly impressive because PSI is almost entirely a volunteer organization, and many of these volunteers are mothers with young children. In 2008, when PSI held its twenty-second annual conference, the organization still had only one full-time employee. Today PSI enjoys broad recognition as a leading resource for laypersons and professionals. PSI promotes awareness and training and "serves over 1,000 callers a month and is staffed by a volunteer team of PSI-trained responders."[21]

There have been other contributions to the rise in public awareness. A number of famous women have bravely come forward to share their stories of postpartum depression, including the actresses Brooke Shields and Marie Osmond, Princess Diana, and the former first lady of New Jersey, Mary Jo Codey. There are now myriad Web sites featuring lesser-known women sharing their stories. Today there is greater awareness and understanding of postpartum depression, and affected women are getting the universal message of PSI: "You are not alone, you are not to blame, there is help and you will feel like yourself again."[22]

But even as the PSI universal message is transmitted to those with depression, the stigma and bias regarding *psychotic* illnesses remains entrenched, and media coverage of it usually pertains to maternal infanticide. The vast majority of women who experience PPP will not hurt anyone and will quickly recover. But it is uncertain whether the universal message of PSI is reaching those with PPP. They too must hear the message: they are not alone … not to blame … [and] there is help and recovery.

Not Alone

This illness is considered rare. But that is not the same as "almost never happens." Usually the rate of occurrence is stated as one to two or one to three out of every thousand postpartum women. (Some speculate that it is even higher.) That is approximately the same rate as Down Syndrome (which affects one out of every 800 babies and is considered one of the most common genetic defects).[23] A recent issue of *Ms. Magazine* stated, "Every minute around the world, 380 women become pregnant."[24] If half of these go to term and one to three out of one thousand develop PPP, it amounts to 273 to 820 new cases of PPP per day. With a 4 percent infanticide rate and a 5 percent suicide rate, that would mean eleven to thirty-three new moms would attempt infanticide daily and fourteen to forty-one would attempt suicide. Women with PPP are indeed not alone.

Although this illness has a long history, it is largely absent in general texts regarding women, regarding madness, and even regarding women and madness. It often seems to be hiding in plain sight in historical accounts. The components are present—recent childbirth and the onset of severe mental illness—but the connection is ignored, and the illness is not named. Without knowledge of others "like them," these women often feel quite alone.

Our myths and media tend to focus on women who have committed infanticide. This does not help sufferers feel less alone, for they are unlikely to want to associate themselves with mothers who kill—or if they do, it is unlikely to be much of a comfort. We need more awareness and acknowledgement of this illness among historians, academics, and members of the press. This must include the fact that infanticide, although a real danger for those with this illness, is rare.

Not to Blame

Postpartum mood disorder advocates have long insisted that women are not to blame for having this illness. Now recent research suggests that PPP may have a genetic cause and that through isolating that gene we may be able to identify those at risk and even prevent cases of PPP.[25]

In modern accounts of maternal infanticide, even those with a strong indication of sudden mental illness, the women are often portrayed as evil and are blamed for the tragedy. How can a woman accept that she is not to blame for her illness when society *does* blame the women who, because of this illness, commit infanticide?

There Is Help

Accounts of infanticide often contain references to help-seeking behavior by the afflicted woman. Of course, all those women who received effective help and did not harm anyone are not covered. This can paint a skewed picture of the efficacy of seeking help, yet this is a crucial message to get out to the public: to encourage and empower these women and their families to seek and to insist upon adequate treatment.

You Will Be Yourself Again

Accounts of postpartum infanticide often ignore the woman's recovery. This is not surprising as many people seem to still believe that mental illnesses are permanent. Furthermore, if the woman's sudden and complete recovery were noted, many people would see that as proof that she was faking or lying. Even in non-tragic cases of PPP, there are few role models of recovery for women with this illness. For many women, part of the recovery from this illness is the recovery from *having had* this illness. This can include learning to trust yourself again, helping your family accept your recovery and regain their trust in you, and believing that you can remain well. We desperately need role models of recovery that these women can point to and say, "She is healthy and well, I too can be healthy and well again." Or, "These women suffered and recovered, I can recover too." These role models can help these women to heal as well as help to dispel the persistent stigma that accompanies this illness.

Of course, if the PPP is linked to an underlying disorder such as bipolar spectrum disorder or schizophrenia, you will still have that disorder, but you will recover from the PPP. In addition, there is beginning to be more information available for expectant mothers with these disorders. I recently learned of a book called *Bipolar and Pregnant: How to Manage and Succeed in Planning and Parenting While Living with Manic Depression* by Kristin K. Finn, which I would expect would have information on avoiding, identifying, and treating PPP. At the 2008 Marcé Society conference, Dr. Philip Boyd presented a paper on mothers with schizophrenia, including a call for more screening and management of this disorder. He reminds us that even mothers with schizophrenia can be helped and can have improved outcomes with proper attention. (He expects to publish a paper on this in the *British Archives of Women's Mental Health* in 2009.) Therefore, women with PPP can be confident that, like all postpartum mood disorders, with proper treatment it will be temporary.

A closer look at our historical literature and current media coverage illustrates the lack of accurate information and understanding of PPP.

HISTORICAL ACCOUNTS OF POSTPARTUM PSYCHOSIS: HIDDEN IN PLAIN SIGHT

Well-educated friends in various professions (nurses, lawyers, feminist educators, doctors, social workers, a paramedic, and a doula) have asked me why they have not heard of PPP until recently. Many of these friends are well read in areas such as women's history, medicine, mental disorders, childbirth, law, and infanticide. I believe they were unaware because in much of the literature on these subjects, postpartum psychiatric illness is hidden in plain sight. Many books that cover these topics and intersections of these topics simply do not make the connection between madness and the postpartum period, even when recounting infanticide.

I noticed this absence of references to PPMDs when reading *Out of Her Mind: Women Writing on Madness*.[26] The preface to the first essay, by Margery Kempe, dated 1436, states that after the birth of a child she went "out of her mind."[27] But the connection is treated as insignificant. I immediately wondered how many of the women in this book became "mad" in the postpartum period. I discovered five descriptions that clearly refer to a woman in the postpartum period. These essays also refer to infants and recent childbirth in an indirect manner—as if they are completely unrelated to the madness.

One of these essays is Charlotte Perkins Gilman's semi-autobiographical classic "The Yellow Wallpaper." I remember reading this essay when I was in college. At the time I had no idea that the illness it described might be brought on as much by childbirth as by social circumstances. I use this essay myself when teaching women's studies, but I have yet to see a women's studies textbook that proposes Gilman may have been suffering from a mental disorder related to childbirth itself.

This connection is not lost on everyone, however. A Wikipedia entry on "The Yellow Wallpaper" states that the madness Gilman describes may be the modern-day PPP. Another Wikipedia entry on Charlotte Perkins Gilman refers to the birth of her daughter Katharine in 1885, and Gilman's "very serious bout of post-partum depression in the months after Katharine's birth." It adds, "This was an age in which women were seen as 'hysterical' and 'nervous' beings, thus, when a woman claimed to be seriously ill after giving birth, her claims were sometimes dismissed as being invalid."[28]

I began searching other books that someone interested in madness, or women, or motherhood, or women and mental health, or women and homicide, might read. The first of these that I picked up was Roy Porter's *Madness, a Brief History.* However, neither childbirth, nor infanticide, nor postpartum illnesses are listed in the index.[29]

Next I read Gail Collins' *America's Women: 400 Years of Dolls, Drudges, Helpmates, and Heroines* which tackles issues of childbearing and insanity—but entirely separately. In many ways this is an excellent book, but she makes no mention of PPMDs or infanticide.

Phyllis Chesler wrote two versions of *Women and Madness.* In the 1972 version, the term "postpartum" is not listed in the index, nor is "postpartum psychosis." The index references to "psychoses (psychotics)" do not lead to any mentioning of PPP. Curiously, the term "postpartum psychosis" *can* be found in the book. It is in a footnote in chapter one in the section on "Heroines and Madness." In describing Dionysus, Chesler states, "It is the child itself which drives the mother mad by its very existence. Just as the child has twice violated the physical boundaries of the mother by its conception and birth, so it drives her to raving infanticide.... In the child-murdering myths of Dionysus one can easily discern some of the underlying ideation of the postpartum psychosis."[30] In her 2005 version of *Women and Madness* Chesler still does not have an index listing for PPP, but again she does mention it. She states, "About 1 to 2 per 1,000 women suffer postpartum psychosis in which they suffer from delusions such as hearing voices that tell them to kill themselves or their infants."[31] No examples are given.

Even Ann Jones' *Women Who Kill* discusses insanity and mental illness but not in relationship to childbearing or infanticide. Maternal infanticide, its punishments *and* motivations are covered in a chapter titled "Foremothers: Divers Lewd Women," but postpartum mental illness is not mentioned as a possible cause. Instead, Jones repeats the motivations often attributed to the women, including bastardy (protecting her reputation, avoiding public shame) and saving the child from a life of servitude. These provide rationales for a woman to choose infanticide. It is interesting that the descriptions of some of these women are consistent with modern understandings of PPP. "Young Alice Clifton, coerced by a white man, seemed to a doctor to have 'lost herself much' in her trouble."[32] On Katherine Garret's execution day, the Reverend Mr. Adams described her as "Stupid & Obstinate and Insensible."[33] Furthermore, "[W]hen first sentenced [Katherine Garret] had been 'thrown into the utmost Confusion & Distress'; she had made 'rash and unguarded' statements and blamed 'all sorts of persons.'"[34] On the gallows she "delivered a memorized prayer, then continued to pray in a 'broken and Incoherent' way."[35]

Without classification it is difficult to say with any certainty whether a *particular* person from the past necessarily experienced postpartum *psychosis*. One online account seems about as certain as they come. It is the account of Sarah Henry, wife of the famous patriot Patrick Henry. On the Web site *Archiving Early America*, Thomas Jewett writes, "At the time Patrick Henry gave his famous speech, few people knew of the personal tragedy that he had been experiencing during the previous three critical years leading up to the Revolution. In 1772, after giving birth to her sixth child, [Edward], Sarah Henry became deeply melancholic and, finally, violent. Henry had her confined to a room in the basement and placed in a strait jacket to prevent her from taking her own life."[36] I have found a few references to Sarah Henry but none that suggest outright that she might have suffered PPP.

Suzanne O'Malley, author of the true crime book *Are You There Alone* about the Yates case, reprinted on her Web site a review of the book by the Journal of the American Medical Association: "'Are You There Alone' demonstrates the paucity of our medical knowledge on childbirth associated mental illness. Accordingly it is an uncommon but excellent teaching tool."[37] What does it say about the coverage of this topic when the *medical* community looks to the "true crime" genre for educational material regarding an illness?

It appears that when postpartum insanity is not the central point of the writing, the link between the postpartum period and mental illness and the link between postpartum mental illness and infanticide or suicide are largely overlooked. The descriptions are there, but the illness itself is hiding in plain sight. Therefore those who are otherwise well versed and well read are less likely to casually come across or become aware of this condition.

HISTORICAL AND MODERN ACCOUNTS OF POSTPARTUM PSYCHIATRIC ILLNESS: SAME AS IT EVER WAS

Historical accounts of PPP do exist. Hilary Marland's *Dangerous Motherhood, Insanity and Childbirth in Victorian Britain* provides many vivid accounts of psychiatric illnesses related to maternity as well as explanations for both the absence of the disorder from records prior to the 1860s and later the "demise" of its recognition as a separate diagnosis.[38] Marland also includes the variety of terms that have been used to refer to this disorder, including: "puerperal insanity,"[39] "puerperal mania,"[40] "puerperal psychosis,"[41] "mania lactea,"[42] "insanity of lactation,"[43] "lactational psychosis,"[44] "mania in childbirth," and "mania furibunda."[45] In spite of this variety of terms, a comparison of historical and modern accounts illustrate the same illness.

Marland noted several themes and described behaviors and statements to illustrate those themes. These themes and the behaviors are still clearly present today. In order to find modern quotes I had to look no further than the first-person stories in this very book. For the purpose of easy comparison, I've designated "DM" for *Dangerous Motherhood* and "UPP" for this book, *Understanding Postpartum Psychosis*, with quotes from UPP in bold type.

Religious Delusions

DM: "I thought a glorious light issued from my temples, and that I was the Virgin Mary."[46]

UPP: **"I was convinced I was the Virgin Mary and I had lived my life on earth as a human"** (Nicole).

DM: A woman claimed to "converse with God."[47]

UPP: **"I had become extremely spiritual ... I felt more 'one' with God than I had ever felt in my life"** (Laura).

DM: "[She] says the devil has got her children & that her soul is lost."[48]

UPP: **"I thought the devil was jumping around from person to person. If someone was talking—the devil was in them"** (Wanda).

Violent and Inappropriate Behavior

DM: "Four days after her first confinement, she became much excited, and at length exceedingly violent, swearing and using most obscene language, although at other times a lady of most correct demeanour."[49]

UPP: A woman who believed her husband was controlled by evil spirits **"began trying to cast these spirits out in the name of Jesus."** Another tried to **"roll the ambulance until it killed all of us"** (Wanda).

Disturbing Delusions and Hallucinations

DM: While in an asylum one woman was the "victim of the most unhappy delusions ... she fancies that the meat she eats is composed of the bodies of her murdered children" who were in fact much alive.[50]

UPP: **"Every time I looked up at the TV, I would see a dagger dripping with blood. I was also hearing a voice say to smother the baby"** (Tara).

DM: Another was "preoccupied and disillusioned, believing that she was to be executed, that she had caused the death of her husband and children."[51]

UPP: **"I was holding my daughter and she looked dead. . . . I couldn't believe that I had killed my whole family!"** (Nicole).

Then, as Now, Women's Delusions Often Involve Their Husband or Others Around Them

DM: "She next began to accuse her friends, especially her husband, whom she charged with infidelity, and an intention to poison her; and it became necessary to separate her from her family. . . . She continued in this state many months, but ultimately recovered, and has had a child since without a recurrence of the disease."[52]

UPP: **"I thought my husband had drugged me,"** and **"I started to think my mom and my husband were evil"** (Wanda).

"I was convinced ... [my husband] had turned the children against me ... I thought everyone was either staring at me or laughing at me" (Nicole).

"I thought that the patients wanted to kill me and that people were hiding in the bushes watching me" (Lisa).

With such detailed historical evidence of this illness, why doesn't this appear in mainstream books—even as a theory? Instead it remains "a condition without an identity." This adds to the misperception that postpartum psychiatric disorders are new or even unreal.

MEDIA: ERRORS, AGENDAS, AND IMPROVEMENTS

Media attention to PPP has been increasing. Online and blog articles that mention PPP are now so frequent that I regularly receive "Google Alerts," sometimes several times a day. (Google Alerts allows a researcher to sign up for notifications when certain terms or phrases appear on the Internet.) Major news outlets have even covered stories of PPP that do not focus on infanticide. I know of at least four. But the most common mention of PPP is in relation to infanticide. I can understand the news value of these tragedies, but imagine if the *only* news coverage of cancer was in relation to persons who have died from it. It would leave little hope for those afflicted with cancer and would add to the stigma that those with terminal illness face. That is the current situation for those with PPP.

Media Response to Maternal Infanticides

Maternal infanticide is unfortunately more prevalent than is commonly believed, but only a few cases grab the attention of the national media. Often those are the most shocking. There may be a rather large number of children involved or the method of killing is particularly gruesome or bizarre, and usually the mother is a person who seems an unlikely candidate for such an act: a high-school student at a prom, a middle-class mother who drives her car into a lake with her children in it, a mild home-schooling suburban mother who drowns her five children. I believe these cases become sensations in part because it is so difficult to understand these tragedies. I believe much of the media—and the public response—is driven by the desire to know *why* it happened, *who* is to blame, and the reassurance that *it cannot happen to us.*

Telling Us What We Want to Hear

Postpartum psychosis cases challenge us, for they deny us easy answers and reassurances. Although there are identifiable risk factors, few doctors do what is necessary to determine if a woman is at risk. We do not fully understand *why* it happens, but we know it is not simply social circumstances. Therefore this illness continues to occur "without warning."[53] This also makes it difficult to place blame on these women. Two prominent authors assert, "It makes no sense to hold someone responsible for a neurochemical event that is out of her control."[54] Our current system does little to train professionals to identify risk factors to prevent this illness, screen women postpartum, or adequately treat these women. Until it does, none of us can be certain that this illness will not touch us—either ourselves or those we love.

Although basic journalism training teaches a reporter the four Ws and an H: *who, what, where, when,* and *how,* journalists often, knowingly or unknowingly, add another W: *why.* It is human nature to want to know *why* something happened, so it is not surprising reporters would want to include it. In addition, reporters frequently not only report events but also interpret them for us. They may feel a *need* to give us the answers to why something happened, identify who is to blame, and thereby reassure themselves and us that we are safe. It is also natural for reporters to be influenced by the culture in which they live. They share our history, myths, and subconscious fears. These may influence a reporter's viewpoint and lead a reporter to fill the gaps with "common knowledge" that is really a common myth. Furthermore it is easier to report common myths than it is to challenge their veracity. This is particularly true when the reporter has a choice of telling us what we want to hear or siding with a mother who has killed her child.

The Need to Know Why

Whenever something bad happens it is human nature to want to know why. Out of this, maternal infanticide and even postpartum psychosis have been blamed on a number of things—such as the woman's character or social circumstances. But what if, as recent research may indicate, it is simply genetic? Consider that as you read the following sections.

"Mad" Versus "Bad"   In *Moving Targets: Women, Murder, and Representation*, Helen Birch states, "[I]n courtrooms and newspapers throughout the Western world, women who kill are divided into two camps: bad—wicked or inhuman; or mad—not like 'ordinary women'."[55] These are tidy little labels that create one-dimensional "others" to explain why something happened. In either case, the label is dehumanizing. Painting someone as wicked or inhumane makes blame and punishment easy. In her book, *Mother Nature*, Sarah Hrdy writes, "Accusing people of depraved behavior can be the first step to viewing them as 'moral inferiors' and denying them basic human rights."[56] If a woman is "evil," we do not have to struggle with our conscience and compassion when meting out punishment.

If a woman is "mad," we do need to bring compassion into the picture. But in the old absolutist view of madness as an inherent and permanent trait, we may forgive them as we permanently lock them away in a psychiatric facility. Our need for compassion itself may be reduced when we tell ourselves that they do not suffer in the same way as the sane, that on some level they are insensitive to their own suffering.

What do we do when we cannot answer the question, "Why?" If the woman is not "bad," but instead her behavior is "unrelated to 'former disposition or habits'"?[57] What if she was mad but unexpectedly and only temporarily? What if she IS an "ordinary woman"? Can we really justify punishment or imprisonment? What is the just and compassionate thing to do?

Bad Social Circumstances   Although experts tend to agree that "[p]ostpartum psychosis is likely of biochemical origin,"[58] many media accounts continue to blame bad social circumstances. Social circumstances, although they may contribute to and exacerbate the problem, do not on their own *cause* PPP. *"Never,* as some of the literature wrongly states, are these conditions solely traceable to the young mother who finds herself immobilized by child care, and because of this becomes upset and ill."[59] (Emphasis in original) Yet time and time again we see references to a woman's circumstances as the reason for the infanticide—or for the illness itself. These ideas are not new. In the nineteenth century, "Some women were seen as more vulnerable by reason of their poverty and want on one hand, or excessive luxury and heightened sensitivity on the other, but the disorder could afflict all women regardless of rank, wealth, geography, marital status, age or childbearing history."[60] It is easy to see how these labels arise out of and perpetuate myths and misconceptions about this illness.

In an article titled "Infanticide is sadly not rare" in *The Gazette* (Montreal), a criminologist at B.C.'s Simon Fraser University refers to the Canadian law on infanticide, stating "[T]he idea was that something about giving birth created the possibility of postpartum depression and therefore made it more likely that women might kill during that first year. . . . The fact that we have that section effectively institutionalizes the possibility that women are subject to some pressures that men are not subject to."[61] The pressures that he notes include women who find childrearing occasionally "frustrating" and "difficult."

This portrayal manages to minimize the illness and the challenges women, particularly marginalized women, face. One might read this and think that these women kill their children because they don't like being inconvenienced. This misogynistic portrayal is similar to some nineteenth-century popular assertions. If a woman was poor, her illness was likely due to financial and social hardships, including overwork. If the woman was wealthy, she was too delicate or nervous for the demands of motherhood or the trauma of birth.

This criminologist further states, "Almost inevitably it has to do with something dysfunctional in the family environment. . . . My guess is that it's probably a family that doesn't have a lot of resources, it doesn't have much of a social network." He does acknowledge, "Of course, a lot of people fall into that category and don't commit those kinds of crimes." Yet that does not lead him to hypothesize that there might be something else going on to distinguish the women who kill from those who do not.

It is unclear why the reporter chose this particular criminologist to interview as it appears that maternal infanticide is not his area of expertise. The criminologist does not refer to any recent literature on the subject but instead makes a "guess."

Unfortunately, misleading articles like this are not rare. Nor are they limited to a focus on poor social circumstances. Much of what passes for "news" about maternal infanticide and about PPP is less than accurate and sometimes less than professional.

The Need to Feel Safe: Not Like Us   Explanations of why a maternal infanticide occurred that utilize characterizations of "mad" or "bad" or blame bad social circumstances serve to distance us from the situation. If I know that I am a good person with no history of mental disorders who enjoys a good social situation—good marriage, planned child, financial security, self-fulfillment—I can rest easy that I could not be one of *those* women. That is what I naively thought before I had my first child. I knew of maternal infanticide. I even knew of the British Infanticide Act. But I believed that *those* women were in abusive relationships, or were young women fearful of strict condemning parents, or drug addicts, or other women who are so desperate that they saw no other solution. *They* were certainly not *me*.

Accurate media coverage of maternal infanticide caused by PPP is likely to cause some concern about who *could* become ill. There are a number of recent articles that are beginning to reflect this concern. In an article posted at NewStateMan (online) the headline asks, "Could you too be a killer mummy?"[62] Yet another reporter observes, "For a new mother, the questions are more stark and more disturbing: Am I capable of hurting my newborn? What could push me over the edge?"[63] This may be the most frightening thing about PPP to the average reader. It is not the thought that some woman might commit infanticide, but rather the fear that *we* or *someone we love* could be *that woman*. This is not a slow deterioration. This is not madness that is brought on by behavior thought of as inherently risky, such as drug use. This occurs to women who do not expect it and did nothing to cause it. And it often becomes severe quickly. This is the uncomfortable reality of PPP in our times.

Yet in spite of the fear that seems to be lurking in the background for many expectant and new mothers and those who love them, I would guess there are few who really *believe* it could happen *to them*.

Randy Gibbs is a founder of "Jenny's Light," an organization to help educate the public about PPP. His sister Jenny committed suicide postpartum and took her little son Graham with her. Randy told me that when Andrea Yates killed her children, prior to his sister's tragedy, he condemned her just as many others did. At the time, he had no idea that *his* family could face a similar tragedy. Unfortunately, Randy is typical. Most of the people I know, myself included, had little concern or sympathy for those with PPP prior to it affecting their lives. We thought it was something that happened to *other people*: people who have something *wrong* with them, people who are fundamentally *not like us*.

PROGRESS AND PERSISTENT PROBLEMS IN THE MEDIA

The abstract for an academic paper, "Singing the 'Baby Blues': A Content Analysis of Popular Press Articles About Postpartum Affective

Disturbances," found that articles about postpartum depression and the baby blues often "contained contradictory information about the definition, prevalence, onset, duration, symptoms, and treatment of postpartum disorders." The authors concluded, "Although the purpose of the articles was to educate readers about an important topic in women's health, they failed to provide accurate information, and thus are not a sufficient resource for new mothers who are seeking to learn about psychosocial aspects of the postpartum period."[64] (While there are numerous articles that reflect cultural biases and prejudices and employ logical fallacies to promote a specific agenda, addressing them is beyond the scope of this chapter. This book is intended for those seeking understanding and accuracy.)

Terminology: Baby Blues or Postpartum Psychosis

The headlines are confusing:

- "Baby blues made me cut my wrists"[65]
- "The Darker Side of the 'Baby Blues'"[66] (The article begins, "Ann Green smothered her firstborn. . . .")
- "'Baby Blues' defense successful in past cases"[67]

In one article with the headline, "Mother kills baby in suicide attempt," the first sentence mentions that the woman may have been suffering from "postpartum depression."[68] Further on the article states: "According to the National Women's Health Education Center, postpartum depression and PPP are serious, treatable mental illnesses that usually affect women within three months of childbirth." This part is good. But then the article continues, "Often called *"baby blues"* the condition is thought to be caused by low levels of certain hormones and can cause new mothers to become irritable, depressed, irrational and even homicidal." Here the reporter has mixed accurate information with *inaccurate* terminology by using the term "baby blues." There are many frustrating examples of this. It is a common mistake. In an article in Slate.com Sally Satel writes: "Our culture uses the terms 'postpartum depression' . . . and 'postpartum psychosis' interchangeably to describe the so-called baby blues."[69] Although I'd agree that these terms are often *used* interchangeably, it is an error to do so. As chapter one of this book illustrates, these are distinct entities. They have different symptoms, different treatments, a different course of illness, and, importantly, different risks.

This confusion over terminology creates a number of problems. Perhaps the two most significant are the potential distress of those 80 percent of women who have baby blues and the 15–20 percent who have depression, thinking their condition could cause them to become homicidal. Conversely, I've heard more than one person, in reference to the

Andrea Yates case, express the sentiment that baby blues and depression don't make you kill your kids; therefore, she must have known what she was doing. Ignorance regarding terminology serves to perpetuate stigma and bias and blocks the route to understanding.

"Wanted to Kill"

Another frequent mischaracterization is that women with PPP *want* to kill their children. It is easy to assume that a woman who has thoughts of killing her child or who believes she must kill her child or whose behavior indicates a deliberate act is someone who *wants* the result. If someone entertains and enjoys occasional thoughts of the freedom of a life without a husband and children it does not mean she *wants* that. I have a single friend who travels extensively and has a fairly glamorous life. Her life is similar to what I once thought mine would be. At times I think it must be nice to live like that. That does not mean I do not love my husband and children. And it certainly does not mean I want to be rid of them.

If a mother believes she must kill her child in order to protect it from a fate worse than death, it does not mean she *wants* the child dead. And if a mother who has intrusive thoughts fears that a part of herself might want to hurt her child, it does not mean she *wants* to hurt the child. It may mean that she has no other way to understand why she is having those thoughts.

Even if a mother says she *wanted* to kill her child because she believed the child was Satan it does not mean that mother wanted her child dead—in her mind it would be Satan that she was killing.

I've never met or read about a woman with PPP who *wanted* to kill her child. Generally I've heard these mothers express it as a need or an absence of feeling or as if something else is controlling their actions, that the act or impulse is not of their own free will.

This may seem a matter of semantics but such representations have a number of negative results. First, for those who come forward and have not committed infanticide, it can be disturbing to think of your child seeing your relationship to him or her represented in that fashion. Second, this error perpetuates the idea that women with PPP kill their children *because they want their children dead*.

In the mid-1800s PPP or mania was described as "typified by the struggle mothers felt between *not wanting to harm* their infants and an inability to prevent themselves from doing so."[70] (Emphasis mine) From a legal perspective, the belief that these women *want* to kill their children can be translated into *malice* and *intent* and as such can justify a charge of first degree murder. Thus this becomes not just a difference of wording, but a description of motive, of state of mind. It is a negation of the plea of insanity. And it is false.

Shading

Slightly different wording can leave a vastly different impression. For example, in the true-crime book *Breaking Point*, police told reporters from the *Houston Chronicle* that Andrea Yates spoke about the killings in a "zombie-like fashion."[71] However, in an online article titled "Mommy Undearest," the author describes Andrea as "calm."[72] Although one might argue that "zombie-like" and "calm" are not so different, they can indicate very different states of mind. Often an article that contains subtle shadings of this nature contains more than a few of them. Issues regarding mental illness, women, crime, and infanticide are sometimes co-opted by people who want to use the story to further their own agenda. Readers, viewers, and listeners should always be on the lookout for logical fallacies, shading of words, and other rhetorical devices that masquerade as truth in the news. Particularly in online sources, but also in major media outlets, these devices can paint a very inaccurate picture while appearing to be straightforward. Although these errors and biases are not always obvious or even intentional, to paraphrase a popular phrase, "Reader beware!"

Grace Awards

Lauren Hale, PSI co-coordinator for Georgia, has created the "Grace Awards" to be awarded quarterly. The following is her explanation of the inspiration for and purpose of these awards:

> The Grace Awards, started in June of 2008, serve to recognize and honor journalists reporting on Postpartum Mood Disorders with dignity, honor, accuracy, and compassion. So many times we read stories in the media about women struggling with PPMDs that not only include inaccurate information, but lack the compassion and dignity these stories deserve no matter how tragic. After reading a few stories with blatant accuracy errors I resolved to do something in order to encourage the media at large to perform their jobs and seek the truth in relation to PMDs. I sincerely hope the Grace Awards grow and serve their purpose.

The Web site for the Grace Awards is http://unexpectedblessing.wordpress.com/grace-awards-for-journalists/.

CONCLUSION

The illness we call "postpartum psychosis" is not new, although it has gone by many names. Yet all names that specifically refer to this phenomenon have been largely omitted from twentieth-century dialogue and literature, including medical and historical literature. When any illness is omitted from our historical accounts, our medical references, and our lexicon, those confronted with that illness suffer unnecessarily.

When this illness is misrepresented in the press, whether deliberately or due to erroneous "common knowledge," the suffering is exacerbated.

Because women and their families remain largely uninformed, those struck with this illness are less likely to anticipate a problem and are, therefore, not prepared. They are less likely to identify the problem, which in cases of PPP can contribute to tragedy.

It is often difficult for these women to find role models of recovery. This can be further isolating and discouraging. The stigma still associated with mental illness keeps many of the women in hiding, even after recovery. When society only knows about PPP through an association with infanticide, the stigma is even harder to face.

The vast majority of women with PPP do not hurt anyone, and their stories are almost completely absent from our popular literature and our media.

It is unconscionable that an illness that has been known as long and in such detail as PPP is still in hiding in our present society. Although dedicated individuals in groups like PSI and the Marcé Society have made phenomenal progress in spite of small numbers and little funding, it is not enough. We need academics, historians, medical professionals, politicians, members of the press, and members of the public, who care about women, children, and families, to educate themselves about this illness. The dark ages of PPP are now. We need to shine the light of knowledge and understanding on this illness. Continuing to ignore it, blaming these women, their husbands, or social circumstances, or reassuring ourselves that these women are "not like us," will not protect our society and will ensure future needless suffering and loss of life.

Perhaps the "Grace Awards" will help to inspire reporters to report on this illness with accuracy and compassion. We need less tolerance for those who intentionally or unintentionally perpetuate negative and inaccurate myths. We need education for all so that the average citizen has enough accurate information to distinguish between common myths and the realities of this illness.

Chapter 4

Legal Views

"When clients come through my office on a daily basis there is a common denominator. Whether it is greed, lust or jealousy ... a lovers' triangle, drugs, money ... there is a baseness, a carnal temptation, a human frailty, that drives them to do what they do. But with Andrea there was none of that. There was no issue other than the upside down world of a mother who loved her children and did what she thought was the very best thing for them. It was a mother's love that was the whole foundation of doing what she did for her children. And she did it FOR her children."[1]

"When a mother harms her child while acting on delusional beliefs, many lives are changed dramatically and permanently. The ignorance of the criminal-justice system further compounds the tragedy."[2]

There is no universal agreement in the United States regarding legal treatment of the mentally ill. This is evident in both civil and criminal cases. All too often the stigmas, prejudices and misunderstandings about mental illness continue to influence judicial decisions. For example, some courts still treat all persons with a history of mental illness as permanently mentally ill. In criminal cases different states have different "tests" for insanity, and some have no "insanity defense" at all.

Even where there are insanity defenses, they are often criticized for having little relation to modern scientific knowledge. A criminal law textbook author observes, "The familiar 'battle of the experts' in insanity trials has embarrassed the [psychiatric] profession enormously by giving the impression that psychiatrists are quacks or worse. But it is the question that the law asks rather than the answers that the experts give that is to blame for the situation."[3] The legal process continues to allow stereotypes, biases, and stigmas to influence the fate of those with a history of mental illness.

The treatment of women who experience PPP is *further* complicated by the confusion in terminology in the medical profession regarding this illness. The official guide to mental disorder classifications, the *Diagnostic and Statistical Manual of Mental Disorders, 4th Edition* (DSM-IV), does not have a distinct diagnosis of "postpartum psychosis." Instead, postpartum mood disorders (PPMDs) are simply recognized as having a "postpartum onset." There is "considerable evidence that postpartum mental illnesses are marked by symptoms peculiar only to them."[4] And there is hope that they will be included in the latest edition, the DSM-V, which is scheduled for release within the next five years.

I asked George Parnham, Andrea Yates's attorney, if he thought having a DSM designation would be helpful. He replied that "DSM recognition of PPP, even if it is not admitted into evidence, is something [the attorneys] could query experts on." He noted that to professionals the DSM is a handbook, "but for the layperson it is a 'bible'—to them it is as close to objectivity about a mental illness as that layperson will ever see."[5] Of course this leads me to wonder if the opposite is true. Does absence from the DSM appear to the jury as *objective truth* that this illness does not exist?

It seems certain that until PPP is recognized as a differentiated diagnosis, women who suffer from this disorder will have a difficult time obtaining justice and a fair trial in the U.S. court system.

These women often face a perfect storm—the confluence of distinct forces that come together to produce tragedy. They suffer a sudden and severe disorder that is often missed or inadequately treated due to a lack of medical recognition. This leads to tragic consequences that are made more turbulent when these women face a legal system where this same lack of DSM recognition leads to a Catch-22 situation. They must demonstrate their actual experience without a recognized diagnosis in a court system that relies on outdated and unscientific approaches to mental illness. Within the legal system they are dependent upon a range of people—from jailers to judges to juries—who are influenced by a society where mental illness is still stigmatized, stereotyped, and misunderstood.

In this chapter, common challenges and biases these women face are highlighted using maternal infanticide to demonstrate the many barriers that must be overcome to obtain fair outcomes. Suggestions for attorneys who assist these women follow. The chapter closes with a brief review of legislation regarding PPMDs. More general issues concerning infanticide, mental illness, and the insanity defense are beyond the scope of this chapter, although they certainly bear upon PPP cases as well.

The injustices that women with this illness face in criminal courts and civil courts have similar causes and characteristics. I have chosen to focus on postpartum maternal infanticide to illustrate these problems.

POSTPARTUM PSYCHOSIS AND INFANTICIDE: THE PERFECT STORM

When a woman has the misfortune of becoming ill with PPP and the added complication of not receiving adequate medical care, having to face an unenlightened legal system creates a "perfect storm" of injustice.

Wikipedia credits the 1997 book *The Perfect Storm* with the origination of the term. It states that this term "refers to the simultaneous occurrence of weather events which, taken individually, would be far less powerful than the storm resulting of their chance combination...."[6] Furthermore, "even a slight change in any one event contributing to the perfect storm would lessen its overall impact."[7]

When a woman with PPP commits infanticide there is often a series of events that, taken individually, would be far less damaging than the tragedy that results from their combination. Furthermore, even a slight change in any one event that contributes to this perfect storm would lessen its overall impact.

INADEQUATE CARE

In cases of PPP many experts have noted that inadequate terminology can lead to inadequate care and inadequate care can lead to tragedy. Ideally women with this disorder would be diagnosed and sufficiently treated—whether for cure or prevention—and tragedies avoided. Until then, it is imperative that the legal system develop more humane processes for dealing with these women. When courts treat maternal infanticide as if each case were a unique and bizarre aberration of motherhood, it does little to encourage the public or the medical profession to become more educated and aware. It allows us to place the blame entirely on the woman. If the legal profession recognized these cases as a failure of medical care, it would provide an incentive for the medical profession to take action to prevent the circumstances that give rise to these tragedies.

Another area of legal involvement is legislation. Legislation can provide for education and research and require that women be offered screening and referrals for adequate treatment. Such legislation is currently pending in several states and in the federal legislature.

PPP is a tragedy for afflicted women and their families. This tragedy can take on horrific proportions in cases of homicide, infanticide, and suicide. Only adequate care can prevent these tragedies. Reforms in the legal system and public education can assist in avoiding tragedy and the re-victimization of these women.

NO LEGAL RECOGNITION OF THE ILLNESS

One possible reform would be an official recognition of PPP by the legal system. There are two significant barriers to this solution. The first is that the legal system tends to rely on the DSM to determine if there is an official diagnosis for a recognized illness. In spite of the fact that there is wide agreement among medical professionals that some women experience sudden and severe psychosis in the postpartum period, without an official designation in the DSM it is more difficult for a court or legislature to justify recognition of the disorder. It is the women who have already suffered unbelievably with this disorder who pay the price of this lack of recognition by the DSM or the courts. "Our reluctance to place [PPMDs] within a diagnostic framework often leads to tragic outcomes for women, families, and society. Moreover, it continues to result in disparate treatment for women in the legal system overall."[8]

The second complication is the fact that our judicial system is actually a number of different, relatively independent legal systems. Each state has its own legislature and its own civil and criminal courts. Accused women face very different standards, rules, and tests for this type of case, depending upon their location. One significant difference is the different tests for criminal insanity. In addition to the insanity test, there are rules affecting pleadings, admission of evidence, and other minutiae that can have a significant influence on a particular case. Obtaining judicial recognition of this illness through legislation would be very difficult and would likely face a constitutional challenge.

Although legislating judicial recognition would be difficult, it is worth considering how legal recognition of this illness might result in a more just and humane outcome. The following are examples of current practices and policies which often result in biased, difficult, or even cruel treatment of these women in today's legal system.

Inhumane Treatment

Women who commit maternal infanticide while experiencing PPP may automatically be viewed by the guards, the therapists, and the prosecutor as alien, unfeeling, and less than human.

Katherine Dillon was clearly mentally ill after the birth of her daughter. After she was arrested for infanticide, she described being put into a strip cell with no clothes, no sanitary pads, no bed, no blankets. Furthermore, "Her food was placed on the floor and the guards made her crawl across the floor to it."[9]

Such treatment is always reprehensible, but it is even more barbaric to treat the mentally ill this way. It is hard to imagine these guards treating a person who has killed another in "self-defense" in a similar manner. If there were legal recognition of this illness, it is likely that a woman in Katherine's position would not be so blatantly revictimized on entry into the legal system.

Prosecutorial Discretion Influenced

"Murder" is a very specific term in our legal system. It requires evidence or proof of a specific state of mind referred to as "mens rea" or "evil intent." It is not enough that a person has committed an act. In our system of justice the moral culpability of the defendant is important. If there is intent, but it is not a *bad* intent, it is not murder. Therefore, self-defense is not murder because the intent to kill was not based on an "evil" or "bad" motive. Similarly, if the person is *incapable* of forming intent (which is an underlying principle for the insanity defense), it is not murder. However, if the prosecutor *presumes* "murder," then the prosecutor assumes evil intent as well.

Wayne LaFave, a legal textbook author, notes that the prosecutor determines "what prosecutions will best serve the public interest."[10] Such discretion suggests that a prosecutor determine the likelihood of moral culpability and the public interest *prior* to charging the defendant. If the prosecutor automatically assumes "murder," when dealing with cases of maternal infanticide, it is unlikely he will use his discretion to consider the influence of PPP. We must ask: Is the prosecution of a woman who killed her own beloved child as a result of a temporary and treatable mental illness likely to further the prosecution's goal to "promote the ends of justice, instill a respect for law, and advance the cause of ordered liberty"?[11]

Ideally all prosecutors would weigh each case on its merits instead of treating all categories of cases the same. But prosecutors who make the assumption that these women are no different from cold-blooded serial killers are more likely to choose to vigorously prosecute and to seek the highest penalty possible *regardless* of evidence of mental illness. If there were a legal recognition of this disorder, prosecutors would take the evidence of PPP into consideration when choosing *whether* to prosecute or in what manner.

Many prosecutors have political ambitions. Some may be influenced by these ambitions to appear 'tough on crime' and uniformly prosecute any homicide. A legal recognition that these women are *temporarily mentally ill* could assist a prosecutor in justifying a more enlightened course of action.

Catch 22: Proving an A-typical Psychosis

Evidence regarding mental health can be "particularly hard to verify."[12] Having a distinct diagnosis is advantageous as elements of a disorder that are difficult to prove, particularly those elements that might be counterintuitive to a jury, can be introduced as possibilities. For example, women who are raped often display a common pattern of response. They often do not appear distraught and delay reporting the rape. Courts now generally allow evidence of Rape Trauma Syndrome to illustrate that these are *common and normal* responses. Without recognition of this syndrome it is difficult for jurors to understand these actions, and so they are likely to base their decision less on the evidence of the rape and more on common myths and pre-existing but erroneous assumptions about what a woman who is raped *would* do.[13] Furthermore, women who are raped often exhibit post-traumatic stress disorder. Yet evidence of this disorder alone would not explain these women's behavior.[14]

Similarly, women with PPP generally must show that they have a recognized disorder. Yet there is no perfect "fit," as they may exhibit symptoms of organic psychosis, schizophrenia, *and* bipolar disorder, or even all three. In addition they often have higher levels of delusions and confusion than women with similar disorders in the general population and often appear to have a waxing and waning of symptoms.[15] Therefore PPP is often considered an "a-typical" psychosis.[16] This leads to the "Catch 22" where the defense counsel may choose to rely on an official diagnostic category such as "organic psychosis" and then persuade the jury that the woman also had symptoms that do not fit well with that category. Either way the defense does not have the advantage of a diagnosis that would convey the unique features of PPP. To make matters worse, the waxing and waning presentation and the temporary duration common to PPP are the opposite of the common myths and assumptions that psychosis would be obvious, constant, and permanent.

Women with PPP today face the same problem rape victims face—the common patterns of behavior and reactions that mark their experience are the very things that make them more unbelievable to those judging them. An attorney representing a rape victim would be at a significant disadvantage if he were barred from showing that his client's reaction is typical. Today a court may bar the *mentioning* of the term postpartum psychosis because it is not an official DSM diagnosis. Furthermore, the prosecution can freely capitalize on erroneous and uninformed assumptions and myths to attempt to *disprove* its very existence!

Just as evidence of Rape Trauma Syndrome helps to combat erroneous myths and establish that there are *usual* hallmarks to this experience, legal recognition of PPP could have the same effect.

Catch 22 Again: Help-seeking Behavior Can Be Used to Discredit Illness

Women with PPP who commit infanticide often have sought help to no avail.[17] Sometimes this failure is due to a misdiagnosis. If a woman erroneously diagnosed with baby blues later attempts to plead insanity based on PPP, the prosecution might use this diagnosis to attempt to discredit the insanity claim because it is widely recognized that baby blues does not lead to infanticide.

Similarly, consider a woman who hears command hallucinations to drown her child. She is fearful and tells her family and her doctor in an attempt to keep her child safe. She is inadequately treated and returned home to care for the child. Shortly thereafter she drowns the child. During her trial the prosecution may seek the death penalty using her help-seeking statements to establish premeditation.

Clearly it is in the interest of society for these women to seek treatment for their illness. It is unconscionable to punish these attempts to find help. Instead we might ask, "Are these the actions of a cold-blooded killer?"

Not Still Insane Can Be a Bad Thing

The insanity defense concerns itself with the defendant's mental state *at the time of the commission of the act*. A person who exhibits mental illness at the time of the *trial* but did not at the time of the act is not a good candidate for the insanity defense. A person who was insane at the time of the act but is well by the time of the trial *is* a candidate for the insanity defense. And there is often a significant lapse of time between act and trial.

Women who suffer PPP often recover quickly and completely. Therefore there is a good chance a woman who experienced PPP will be well by the time of her trial. These women often face the skepticism that anyone using the insanity defense is likely to face—the belief that they are trying to fool the court.[18] The jury may therefore scrutinize the defendant carefully to determine if she appears sane. A woman who had psychosis may not only appear sane, but also she may in fact *be* sane. A skeptical jury may, consciously or unconsciously, regard the defendant's sanity as proof that she *was not* insane at the time of the act. This is particularly true of jury members who believe that all mental illnesses are permanent. If there were legal recognition of PPP, the temporary nature of this illness would be easier to establish to disabuse the jury of their erroneous preconceptions of mental illness.

Expert Witnesses: Not Required to Be Expert in Reproductive Mental Health

Both the defendant and the prosecution rely on expert testimony. These experts are not impartial, however. It is fairly easy for each side to hire an expert or experts whose testimony will match their agenda. Therefore, the contradictory testimony of the "experts" may do little to inform the jury.

Furthermore, these "experts" do not have to be experts on PPP—or even on PPMDs—or even on women's reproductive mental health! In addition, they may not see women with PPP in their practice—if they have a practice. Finally, they might have *no* specific experience *or* training on *postpartum* maternal mental health.[19] If there were legal recognition of this disorder, it would be more likely that experts would be required to have had training or to at least have familiarity with current research in the field.

Not Viewed in Context

In the case of maternal infanticide,*"Each act is judged in isolation, with little or no regard for similar cases."*[20]

What if every defendant in a self-defense case had to prove not only the self-defense itself but also the concept of self-defense? In essence, that is what lack of medical and legal recognition of PPP requires. Instead of demonstrating that these women are part of "a recurring pattern of the destruction of planned-for, wanted children by their own mothers,"[21] each one is treated as a shocking aberration. Without this recognition jurors might well wonder, "If there *is* an illness that can cause a good mother to kill a child she loves while temporarily ill, why aren't there *other* women like this defendant?"

Don't Tell the Jury

Generally juries are not told what the different outcomes of their verdicts might be. For example, a defendant found not competent to stand trial does not necessarily go free. That person will likely be held in some form or incarcerated until the time that she is competent. Similarly, if a defendant is found "guilty but insane" or "not guilty by reason of insanity," it does not mean the defendant walks out of the courtroom a free person. She is likely to be confined in a mental institution until she is determined to be well enough to re-enter society without being a risk to society. Although such knowledge may persuade a jury to be more compassionate if they believe the defendant to be mentally ill, courts generally do not allow the defense to inform the jury of these potential outcomes.

No Easy Solution

How are these women viewed in other countries? "The general trend in Britain, Canada and several European nations is to treat these cases as instances of mental illness. The British Infanticide Act of 1938, for example, authorizes leniency for a woman convicted of killing her own child under the age of twelve months."[22] This act essentially dictates that a woman who kills her infant, upon showing that "the balance of her mind was disturbed," will not be charged with more than manslaughter.[23] Some find even the British law too narrow and unjust.[24] In Sweden they now use a panel of doctors to determine the outcome in these cases.[25]

In the United States creation of an official designation of leniency for these women is problematic as criminal law is generally formulated by states. Having a separate system of courts might be too cumbersome. Perhaps there could be some compromise. Many family courts now refer cases to mandatory mediation because mediation provides an opportunity to manage these cases in a healthier way than the win/lose nature of traditional litigation. Similarly, criminal courts might refer such cases to a panel of medical doctors to determine whether there is a more efficient, effective, and humane method of processing them.

A Note About Civil Courts, Yet Another Catch 22

In criminal court a woman may be barred from introducing evidence of "postpartum psychosis" to illustrate that her act and state of mind were consistent with those of other women who suffer from this illness. In civil courts such evidence is admissible—often, however, to her detriment. "Since rules of evidence are typically less strict in civil courts, postpartum syndromes are readily admitted into evidence during civil proceedings, where this evidence is almost always used in opposition to a woman's interests."[26] For example, the woman's history of PPP may be used to portray her as an unfit mother.

On the other hand, if courts recognize that women may be emotionally unstable after pregnancy but *do not* recognize the realities of the spectrum of postpartum illnesses, the door is open to stigma, bias, and ignorance. Dr. Spinelli cites an example from the 1997 Tennessee appellate court regarding a biological mother who, in an attempt to reverse an adoption decree, claimed postpartum illness rendered her incompetent to consent to the adoption. The court stated, "We do not dispute that [the mother] was probably depressed or emotionally distraught following this rather traumatic experience, but it is not unusual for there to be depression and distress following the birth of a child, even under the best of circumstances. If emotional distress meant that a parent was always incompetent to consent to an adoption, we would rarely have adoptions in this state."[27]

This court decision echoes the old stereotype that women's reproductive events render them mentally incompetent. In essence the court is saying that all women are emotionally distraught after childbirth *always to the same degree*, and therefore the emotional distress of a particular mother is either inadequate to establish incompetence or *new mothers are always incompetent*. This type of false dichotomy is and has historically been a method of reducing women to one-dimensional stereotypes.

This decision is doubly damaging considering there are people who currently oppose postpartum psychiatric designations or even education and screening for these disorders. Given the continuing discriminations and injustices based on prejudicial and outdated views of women, that opposition is somewhat understandable. But it leaves in place a system that does a disservice to women who *do* have emotional disorders in the postpartum period or that are otherwise related to reproductive events. We should not sacrifice our sisters to our fears of sweeping generalizations and renewed bias. We should stand up to these false-hoods and demand that women be treated as more than these one-dimensional stereotypes.

Recognition of the full spectrum of PPMDs could help to discredit comments like that of the Tennessee court. Instead of painting all women as equally "emotionally distraught" the court would be faced with distinguishing between the capacities of women with baby blues versus a woman with a severe postpartum illness.

ARCHAIC, UNPREDICTABLE, AND UNSCIENTIFIC INSANITY LAWS

There are a number of problems with today's insanity laws—from overzealous prosecutors to legal and medical standards that are in-compatible. Insanity is a particularly messy area of law. It attempts to apply rational standards to something that is, by its very nature, irra-tional. Consider the woman who abandons her infant in a parking lot and then goes to a police station to turn herself in and to alert the police to rescue the child. Is her act rational because it affects the res-cue of the child? Is it irrational because she could have just brought the child to the police? Does it prove she knew what she did was wrong? What if she immediately asks the police to return the infant to her? How does that impact our view of her mental state? I believe Dr. Spinelli put it well, "The danger ... is that you may be applying sanity to insanity—applying rationality to the irrational thoughts."[28]

I realize that creating and enforcing insanity laws justly is inherently difficult. But in cases of PPP, justice is harder to obtain due to societal views and expectations of motherhood, the passions these cases arouse, existing stigmas, and, once again, lack of recognition of this illness.

Inconsistent Application

Even the same test for insanity can result in vastly different verdicts. Theoretically one purpose insanity tests serve is to have an impartial standard to protect the truly insane from the inflamed passions of soci-ety—modern-day mob justice. But the variations in verdicts under the same test suggest these tests are less than impartial. Their application indeed seems a modern variation of mob justice—where the passions of the community, not the condition of the accused, determine how the

test is applied. Consider this quote by the eminent U.S. Supreme Court
Justice Benjamin Cardozo in 1915:

> A mother kills her infant child to whom she has been devotedly attached.
> She knows the nature and quality of the act; she knows that the law con-
> demns it; but she is inspired by an insane delusion that God has appeared
> to her and ordained the sacrifice. It seems a mockery to say that, within
> the meaning of the statute, she knows that the act is wrong. If the defini-
> tion propounded by the trial judge is right, it would be the duty of a jury
> to hold her responsible for the crime. We find nothing either in the history
> of the [M'Naghten] rule, or in its reason or purpose, or in judicial exposi-
> tion of its meaning to justify a conclusion so abhorrent.[29]

Cardozo used this as an example of a defendant who would be
clearly incapable of understanding the moral wrongness of her action.
Yet there are women similar to the one in this example, tried by a
court applying the M'Naghten standard (explained below), who have
been found responsible and now reside in prison. Women like this
may face a life sentence or even the death penalty.

Medical and Legal Standards Are Different

For a woman with PPP, it is *not* enough that she prove she was psychotic. At the 2008 Postpartum Support International Conference, key-
note panelist George Parnham, attorney for Andrea Yates, illustrated
this point by showing a picture from *USA Today* with the headline
"'Psychotic', but is Andrea Yates legally insane?" The reason proving
psychosis is not sufficient is that a person who has severe psychosis
may not meet that state's test for legal insanity. She must show she can
meet the test for insanity (which varies by state). Generally the defense
must prove that the defendant either did not know her act was
"wrong" or could not control herself.

Modern medical standards and definitions of mental illness often
bear little resemblance to the legal tests for insanity. Juries face medical
experts advising them in terms that have little to do with the legal test
they must apply or medical experts who testify in terms that meet the
legal language but have little relation to the understandings, definitions, and terms utilized by their profession. In some cases, a layperson
in the jury is asked to apply legal standards to a medical condition
where the definitions of the law and those of medicine are different
between the professions *and* contested *within* the professions.

Different Jurisdictions, Different Outcomes

Different jurisdictions in the United States have different laws.
Therefore two women with almost identical circumstances may have

extremely different outcomes. "[A] woman who receives a prison sentence in one state could receive the death penalty in another, despite the identical circumstances of the crime."[30] This may be influenced by a number of factors: the amount of publicity a case gets, the police characterization of the woman and the scene of the incident, the prosecutor's knowledge of this illness, the evidence rules in that jurisdiction, the judge and jury's understanding and familiarity with this illness, the ability of the woman to pay for legal costs, the insanity law in that jurisdiction, and the method in which it is applied. These are some of the factors that can influence the outcome *apart from anything about the woman as an individual.*

The two tests for insanity that are most widely used in the United States today are the M'Naghten test and the Model Penal Code test. A brief history of these tests illuminates why they are often criticized as being too narrow and unscientific for the requirements of justice.

The M'Naghten Test

The M'Naghten test was used—and widely discussed—in the case of Andrea Yates, the Texas woman who drowned her five children in 2001. It basically states that the defendant must prove that she was laboring under such a defect of reason, from a disease of the mind, as to not know the nature and quality of the act she was doing, or to not know what she was doing was wrong. This is often referred to as the "knowledge of right and wrong" test or the "knowing" test.

Creation of the M'Naghten Test
In Britain in 1843, Daniel M'Naghten was accused of attempting to assassinate the prime minister of England. At that time the courts used a sixteenth-century test that was essentially the same as the current-day M'Naghten test. But in this case, the progressive court looked to the emerging scientific understanding of insanity and determined that the old "knowledge of right and wrong" test was too narrow to address the complexities of mental illness. Daniel M'Naghten was found "not guilty by reason of insanity."

This verdict enraged Queen Victoria, who had faced three assassination attempts herself. She summoned the judges of the common law courts and instructed them to clarify the insanity defense. Not surprisingly, given the apparent wishes of the Queen, the judges revived the old sixteenth-century test. Ironically, this is now known as the "M'Naghten test"—named after the very case that rejected it in favor of a more enlightened, scientific understanding of insanity.[31]

Criticisms of the M'Naghten Test
The United States inherited the British common law—including the M'Naghten test for insanity. Not

surprisingly, this test, regarded as unscientific even at the time of its adoption, has received significant criticism. In addition to being unscientific, M'Naghten has been widely criticized for being too narrow (for focusing only on cognition, not ability to control behavior), for usurping the function of the jury (by limiting the basis of its decision to this test as opposed to weighing the evidence to determine if its members believe the defendant lacks actual culpability), and for being too simplistic (failing to recognize degrees of capacity and the complexity of mental illness).

This test is particularly problematic in cases of PPP infanticide. After all, how can the concept of "knowing" apply to a woman who "is urged on by some unaccountable impulse to commit violence on herself or on her offspring, while at the same time being impressed with horror and aversion at the crime"?[32] Or what of the mother who knows it is legally wrong to kill her child but also in her delusion "knows" it is necessary to save its very soul, even if it means sacrificing her own?

Park Dietz was the prosecution's mental health expert in the Andrea Yates case and the only expert out of a dozen to determine she was sane.[33] Later Dietz testified on behalf of Deanna Laney, another Texas woman who killed her children, whom he found to be insane. Both women were delusional and heard voices. The difference between the two cases, in Dietz's opinion, was the *moral authority* of the voices they heard. Laney heard God telling her to kill her children while Yates heard Satan speaking to her. Deitz determined that because God is a recognized moral authority, Laney did not know what she was doing was *wrong* and so was insane according to M'Naghten. But because Satan is not a recognized moral authority, Yates knew what she was doing was wrong, and therefore was not insane according to M'Naghten.[34] He determined this even though he also knew Yates claimed she did what she did in order to save her children. Using this analysis it did not matter if Yates believed she was saving the souls of her children. It did not matter if she believed it was the right thing to do. It did not matter if she believed she would be arrested and put to death and that her death would free the world from Satan. It did not matter that she was hearing voices and had a history of mental illness. It could be argued that under M'Naghten she knew the nature and quality of her act (that her children would die) and, according to Dietz, *because Satan is not a moral authority*, she knew what she was doing was wrong and therefore was not insane.

M'Naghten has provoked strongly worded criticism. In 1930, "Mr. Justice Cardozo observed that 'everyone contends that the present definition of insanity has little relation to the truths of mental life.'"[35] So why haven't we moved away from such an outdated, unscientific, simplistic test? Perhaps it is the very lack of complexity that makes it so appealing. Do we find mental illness so threatening and difficult to understand that we are willing to sacrifice justice for simplicity?

The Model Penal Code Test (or ALI Test)

Around 1953, in recognition of the serious flaws and unscientific basis for the M'Naghten test, the American Law Institute (ALI) began to formulate a more modern test for insanity. This test was adopted as Section 4.01 of the Model Penal Code (MPC) in 1962. Known as the MPC or ALI insanity test, it was adopted by many courts as it was widely recognized to be superior to the M'Naghten test. This test states: "A person is not responsible for criminal conduct if at the time of such conduct, as a result of mental disease or defect, he lacks substantial capacity either to appreciate the wrongfulness of his conduct or to conform his conduct to the requirements of law."[36]

Although there was acknowledgment that this, or indeed any legal standard, would be difficult to justly apply in all cases, it was still seen as a vast improvement over M'Naghten. In his concurrence in *U.S. v. Freeman*, Circuit Judge Waterman noted that future expert understanding of mental illness may require further judicial correction or improvement to this test.[37]

Return to the M'Naghten Test

In 1981, John Hinckley Jr. attempted to assassinate then-President Reagan. He succeeded in shooting the president and several of his aides, including the severely wounded press secretary, James Brady. There was no doubt that Hinckley did it, as the shooting was captured on camera. In 1982, Hinckley was found "not guilty by reason of insanity" and confined to a mental institution. The nation was stunned. Once again a sensational, politically charged trial provided impetus to turn back the clock. The more enlightened approach of the MPC fell out of fashion, and the M'Naghten test again became the standard for many courts.

This move away from a scientifically based standard is not a matter of semantics. Dr. Margaret Spinelli asserts, "Defendants with mental illness who face the criminal justice system have the right to a defense based on scientific fact. Such a defense is essential for equal representation under the law."[38]

Legal recognition of PPP would help to ensure equal representation for these most unfortunate women.

CULTURAL PERCEPTIONS INFLUENCE TRIAL OUTCOMES

Who are the people who determine what should happen to a woman who commits maternal infanticide? The prosecutor plays a role, as does the judge. And of course, so does the jury—members of the public. We are all influenced by the culture we live in. Although the profession of psychiatry has progressed enormously since the days of phrenology (studying the shape of the skull to determine mental illness), the public perception of the field has not kept apace. When I interviewed Dr. Margaret Spinelli for this book, she commented, "Courts still feel [we] are coming in and presenting Freud. This is science ... not Freud. Juries need to understand this."[39]

In the United States there is also a strong stigma regarding mental illness. In her tragicomic autobiographical novel, *Hillbilly Gothic*, Adrienne Martini discusses the reasons it is difficult to find historical accounts of postpartum mental illness. "First, history has a tendency to ignore women in general unless they do something spectacular or globally noteworthy.... Second and perhaps most important, madness tends to be shoved under the rug because it is so stigmatized.... Third, and perhaps the aspect we talk about the least, is that most crazy people are scary to the outside observer, objects of fear and derision rather than compassion."[40] There is also a romanticized view of motherhood. "Because the new mother is expected to be unfailingly happy, the stigma of mental illness is even more pronounced at this time in a woman's life."[41] In her book *Misconceptions* Naomi Wolf refers to the modern childbearing experience and introduction to new motherhood as "almost a recipe for postpartum depression," and states, "much of the typical birth experience is crazy-making."[42] She too recognizes the less than realistic view of motherhood, stating, "[i]f women are surprised to experience more difficulty than they were prepared for, it is because they are given the wrong expectations."[43]

One barrier to educating the public is the attitude that negative perinatal experiences should be kept under wraps to keep from scaring new mothers. But what about the woman who becomes ill? It is very scary to have a severe postpartum mood disorder and not know effective treatments are available. This ignorance has ramifications beyond the individual. When public awareness centers on women who have committed infanticide, evidence and claims of mental illness may look self-serving. A woman who committed infanticide may be characterized as "bad," if she displayed anger or irritation, was slovenly about her housework, or expressed ambivalence about having a child. But these are all potentially *normal* behaviors. Conversely, if a new mother stays up all night cleaning the house, is always on schedule, very talkative, well coifed, and immaculately dressed with a clean, neatly dressed baby, it does not trigger the concern that there may be mania present, for there is an expectation that all new mothers *could* do that with little effort.

These outdated views of psychiatry, stigmas related to mental illness, and romanticized view of motherhood all contribute to the likelihood that the jury will be predisposed to condemn a woman who has killed her child, whether she is mentally ill or not.

WHAT IS THE RESULT OF THIS PERFECT STORM?

The legal system in the United States today virtually guarantees that a woman who encounters the legal system due to PPP is likely to face unnecessary bias and ignorance. There is significant risk that her treatment will be anything but fair.

Just like a hurricane, this illness can devastate the homes of the wealthy and the poor. It does not spare the virtuous or the educated. Some are more at risk than others, although they might not know it. Some may be better able to find help to assist their recovery. And some will be destroyed before they are even aware what is happening.

Those who must face the legal system are often devastated by the primary storm only to then be repeatedly, brutally battered by the aftermath. Instead of receiving lifeboats they are told they should not have been there—as if their presence there were a choice. Instead of food supplies they are told they deserve to starve.

A woman may be, up to the onset of the illness, a good and loving mother. She may then suddenly become ill and kill because of PPP. She may then recover and be no threat to anyone. Yet she may be imprisoned for life or even receive the ultimate penalty. She didn't choose to do wrong; she was not a bad person. She did not cause or choose her illness. She likely sought help but was failed by those who were supposed to care for her—who might have even missed the opportunity to prevent the illness itself. Furthermore, she is grieving the unbearable burden of the loss of her child.

DEFENSE ATTORNEYS IN POSTPARTUM PSYCHOSIS INFANTICIDE CASES

If the medical system fails to save these women from the storm of psychosis, their best hope of being spared total destruction may be in finding a knowledgeable and competent defense attorney. Yet even then the woman may face challenges. It may be difficult to quickly find a competent and willing attorney. If the attorney is unfamiliar with the unique features of PPP, he is very likely to miss important opportunities to preserve important evidence and make the best case for his client. There may be delays in finding qualified experts. These delays could quite literally cost the woman her life.

An Interview with George Parnham, Andrea Yates's Attorney

George Parnham is probably the most famous defense attorney for a woman with PPP—Andrea Yates. I interviewed him about his experience defending Yates and his advice for other defense attorneys. The following is based on that interview.

It is in Parnham's nature to empathize with his clients and want to help them, not only legally, but also in finding resources to get well. But even this empathetic, experienced criminal-defense attorney had difficulty facing this woman who had killed her five children. "I couldn't connect the dots," Parnham said. "It defies the very concept of motherhood." He understood how the community could be "so unified in their hatred of this mother." In his frustration he spoke with a counselor. The counselor asked him if he believed Yates was ill. Parnham said he did. Even the legal and medical experts of the State of Texas did. The counselor asked him if he believed Yates loved her children. He did. "The bottom line is," reports Parnham, "if you believe she was mentally ill and believe she loved her children then you realize what she did was a supreme act of love for her kids—in her psychotic, delusional state."[44]

Parnham went from not being able to identify with his client to seeing her as a whole person. He now describes her as "good, sweet, kind, caring." Although it is not unusual for criminal law attorneys to genuinely care about their clients, it is unusual for them to continue to speak out and work to educate others because of a case. But that is what Parnham did. He now helps to educate the medical and legal communities about PPP. It is not imperative for all these attorneys to become activists, but we do need a way to quickly connect women in this situation with willing and educated attorneys. There is much for them to know, and one of the most crucial aspects in representing any woman in a case arising from PPP is that of timing.

An attorney representing one of these women must find a psychiatrist who specializes in women's mental health (and understands PPP) as quickly as possible. "If postpartum psychosis truly is present," advises Parnham, "get a video camera and an expert witness and interview the client as soon as possible." This is crucial to preserve evidence of her psychosis because these women can recover functioning so quickly. Parnham learned this the hard way. "I did not appreciate how quickly symptoms may disappear," he says.

Parnham also advises: become acquainted with DSM terminology, use an expert to educate yourself, and become intimately familiar with the insanity definition in your jurisdiction. "Lastly, when interpreting your client's actions," Parnham states, "lose your objectivity and see her action through her own eyes and not the eyes of an observer." He compares this to self-defense where it is not necessary that the person was *in fact* in danger of being killed *but believed* she was and had reason to believe that.

Parnham advises other attorneys to "resist the temptation of being repulsed by your client's actions." It is his appreciation of this subjective view that enabled Parnham to understand that what Yates did was done *for* her children.[45]

Parnham now understands the unique features of this illness and the importance of quickly obtaining counsel and securing evidence. Delays can do irreparable harm, and the woman's very life is probably at stake. However, just the process of finding willing counsel may create an unnecessary delay. Therefore, Parnham believes there is a need to have a list of willing attorneys in every jurisdiction, preferably who are already educated about PPP. If a woman could immediately connect with an attorney who knows the steps to take and experts to call, it could make a significant difference in the success of the case.

Defending Postpartum Psychosis: A Game Plan

1. Work with an expert.
2. Gather evidence in a timely fashion.
3. Understand the illness.
4. Gather evidence of the pre-pregnancy, pre-birth personality.
5. Be able to "get inside" the client's head and understand her experience so thoroughly as to be able to show a jury or judge.

The first step is finding a qualified expert. Contacting experts in the field, both for understanding and to assist in the trial, is a necessity. This should be done as soon as possible to better understand the client and how to help her. Ideally the attorney would already be familiar with one or two experts in maternal mental health who would present well to a jury. "It is very important for psychiatrists working with a defense team to be able to talk with a jury and provide the jury with underlying physiology of pregnancy and postpartum and how hormones affect the brain."[46]

Second, immediately secure evidence of the client's illness. Timing is crucial. Experts often stress that it is important to have the woman examined by psychiatric professionals *as soon as possible* as women tend to rapidly recover from this illness and the defense may be left with little medical evidence of the psychosis.[47]

The third step is learning to understand the illness. There are a number of written resources as well as organizations that can help, Some are listed in the appendices of this book. This is important in framing the approach to the case and the case itself.

The nature of this illness makes the past personality and habits of the woman particularly significant. Therefore it is important that the attorney examine the "pre-pregnancy, pre-birth personality."[48] This includes gathering evidence from old acquaintances, school friends, and work associates, as well as documents such as school records and teacher evaluations.[49] These can be used to illustrate that the character and behavior of the woman was of a nature so contrary to the act of infanticide as to strain the imagination.[50] Finally, an attorney must really listen to the client. The attorney should try to understand her experience from her perspective while incorporating knowledge of her pre-pregnancy personality. What did she think was happening? What were her motives for her actions? Did she understand the consequences of her actions? If she hurt the child, did she know what she was doing would ultimately harm the child? If so, did she do it to serve a greater purpose? Consider this: if what the client believed happened or would happen was real, would there be a way to understand her actions in light of her pre-pregnancy personality? For example: if she was a loving mother, why might a loving mother act as she did?

Other Considerations for Defense Attorneys

In addition to these subjective observations, there are other factors which may indicate a mother was likely suffering from psychosis, if they are understood in the context of the illness:

1. *No history of child abuse*. It is not unusual for there to be no history and no evidence of child abuse in these cases. These women are not abusive mothers whose violence eventually escalates to the level of homicide. Although women who are abusive certainly can become psychotic, abuse is not a hallmark of PPP infanticide cases.

2. *Reporting homicidal thoughts to medical authorities ahead of the act*. This is not an indication of premeditation. Women who report these thoughts often are disturbed by them and *do not* wish to act upon them. They report these thoughts in order to prevent or avoid the outcome.

3. *Already seeking or receiving medical help*. Unfortunately, a woman in this situation may not have received an adequate diagnosis or treatment, even if she sought it.

4. *Making no attempt to hide their crime*. In fact, many of these women are the first to call 911 or report their crime to the police. This does not prove that the woman knew her act was wrong. Due to the waxing and waning aspect of this illness, her state of mind at the time of the act and directly after the act may be significantly different. A woman who calls 911 may be sincerely seeking help and may not even realize that she was the cause of the emergency. Also, some of these women may understand that what they are doing is legally wrong but cannot stop themselves. Or they may believe it is *morally* right.
   This does not mean that a woman who does not report her crime or who seeks to hide her involvement is NOT suffering PPP. Mental illnesses, including PPP, are not truth serums. People suffering these illnesses may lie.

5. *Bizarre behavior*. Often these women do or say bizarre things unrelated to the homicide. If we are paying attention, this gives us an opportunity to act and prevent tragedies. Unlike women who lash out in a moment of fury and kill their children, women with PPP who kill their children

often exhibit strange behavior long before the tragic act. If we understand that strange behavior postpartum may signal a risk to mother and child, we have an opportunity to intervene.

6. *Logical planning, illogical reasoning.* Although some seem to believe that if a woman acts deliberately or makes plans she cannot be insane, in fact, many women who suffer from PPP illustrate a mix of rational and irrational thought. Again, Andrea Yates is an example: she did not act until she was alone in the house with the children. She locked the doors and filled the tub and began to kill her children one by one. She did the logical things a person who is determined to kill would do. It is hard to understand that a woman acting so deliberately could not stop herself. But that is indicative of asking the wrong question. She did not choose to stop. She chose to kill her children. It is the *why* that is illustrative. She felt she *had to* or they would be doomed to eternal damnation. Her actions were based on delusional beliefs.

7. *Previous suicide attempt.* Researchers Meyer and Oberman observed that "... mothers who attempt suicide and then resort to infanticide pose a greater risk to all or the majority of their offspring."[51] These mothers may attempt suicide in order to prevent harming their children. These suicide attempts are another example of a lost opportunity for diagnosis and prevention.

Furthermore, it is not just criminal-defense attorneys who can benefit from understanding these features of PPP. These may arise in custody cases, divorce cases, guardianship cases, discrimination cases, and others. Just as the medical community needs a better understanding of PPP if these women are to receive adequate care, the legal community must be educated as well if these women are to receive fair and equal treatment under the law.

LEGISLATION

Although we have noted that national legislation requiring legal recognition of PPP would be extremely difficult to achieve, legislation can be effective in other ways. Legislation seeking to require and/or fund screening, training, treatment, education, outreach, and research can have a significant impact on preventing the personal and societal ravages of this illness.

There are a number of state and federal legislative initiatives that have been passed or are pending. Many of these seem to have been directly influenced by tragedy. Some examples of state legislation are:

New York: In 1998 New York State Senator Hugh Farley, a republican from Schenectady, sponsored "New York State Public Health Law 2803-J, which was the "[c]ountry's first public health law requiring that all hospitals and birthing centers provide information on postpartum depression." This legislation followed the postpartum suicide of one of Farley's staff members.[52]

California: Postpartum Support International (PSI) has long supported legislation to help women with PPMDs. One of PSI's early victories was California State Resolution #23 in 1989, which "was passed to raise the level of competence of local corrections and probations officers about postpartum psychosis." This legislation was in reaction to an infanticide.[53]

Texas: In September of 2003, Texas House Bill 341, "also known as the Andrea Pia Yates Bill" (after the Texas woman who drowned her five children in 2001), passed. It requires that perinatal healthcare providers provide their patients with information on resources for counseling.[54] However, in 2007 the Texas Legislature failed to pass H.B. 2964 and H.B. 1388, which sought to require mental health services for women diagnosed with postpartum depression up to one year after giving birth. This legislation followed four high-profile cases of postpartum maternal infanticide with evidence of a mood disorder that resulted in the deaths of ten Texas children.[55]

New Jersey: In 2006 New Jersey passed the "Postpartum Depression Law," which became "the first in the country to require all healthcare providers to screen women who have recently given birth for postpartum depression and to educate women and families."[56] The law was introduced by State Senate President Richard Codey, whose wife, Mary Jo Codey, suffered severe postpartum depression.

Federal: There is also federal legislation pending, commonly referred to as the MOTHERS Act (Mom's Opportunity to Access Health, Education, Research and Support for Postpartum Depression). This was first introduced during the 109th Congress, second session of the Senate, in July of 2006 as Senate Bill 3529 by Senators Robert Menendez (D-NJ) and Richard Durbin (D-IL).[57] It has many provisions similar to the New Jersey state law and incorporates the Melanie Blocker Stokes Research and Care Act, which is explained below.[58] On October 15, 2007, this bill, now called "The Melanie Blocker Stokes MOTHERS Act," passed in the House with bipartisan support. Although recently smeared by some bloggers as a bill pushed by "Big Pharma," this bill is actually the result of the work of dedicated individuals who have been personally touched by postpartum illness, grassroots and advocacy organizations such as PSI and The Children's Defense Fund, and a number of medical professional organizations such as the American College of Obstetricians and Gynecologists.

The original Melanie Blocker Stokes Postpartum Depression Research and Care Act (HR20) was introduced and sponsored by Congressman Bobby Rush (D-IL). This legislation, named after Melanie Blocker Stokes, who committed suicide due to PPP, was first introduced in 2001. Melanie's mother, Carol Blocker, has been a staunch advocate for this legislation "so others will be spared the tragedy she and her family have experienced."[59] Melanie's story appears as a chapter later in this book.

Unfortunately on July 29, 2008, the Melanie Blocker Stokes MOTH-ERS Act, which was rolled into the "Advancing American Priorities Act," failed to pass in the Senate. However, activists for women with these illnesses are still hopeful. In an email forwarded to members of PSI, Susan Stone, former president of PSI, heralded the good news that the inclusion in the "Advancing American Priorities Act" raised aware-ness and generated "unprecedented coverage by major press agencies resulting in even more attention and awareness of the need for its criti-cal initiatives for mothers, infants and families." Stone, noting that the act was not *defeated*, calls the MOTHERS Act a "no brainer" bill and calls for the preparation for the next presentation of this act "with a growing force of American families who have waited too long and long enough." And, I would add, with the force of all those families in the future who will face postpartum illness with a different level of knowledge, care, and support after this bill is passed.

CONCLUSION

Whether or not the initial decision to omit PPP from the DSM was correct, the result has been that this illness has been treated, not as a version of another illness, but as if it does not exist. In spite of the fact that psychotic illness following childbirth is recognized as a risk, the absence of terminology contributes to an uninformed public, and inad-equate treatment and monitoring for those afflicted.

The legal arena is also affected. "Limited diagnostic guidelines," asserts Dr. Margaret Spinelli, a leading researcher, author, and clinician in this field, "leave sentencing and treatment decisions in the hands of the U.S. courts with little or no contribution from psychiatry."[60]

Where modern scientific knowledge has little room, old biases and stereotypes seem abundant for filling the gaps. Public ignorance, failure by medical providers, and continuing bias against and stereotyping of the mentally ill create a "perfect storm" for those unlucky women who face our criminal law system due to PPP.

Tornados are infamous for destroying one house and leaving a neighboring house untouched—or destroying all but one house on a block. The difference is a matter of luck. If a woman is unlucky enough to face the "perfect storm," her outcome is largely dependent on luck. Is she lucky enough to have a talented attorney who is educated (or interested in becoming educated) about PPP? Is she lucky enough to be in a state with a more modern approach to the insanity defense? Do those she must face—the police, examiners, guards, court personnel, judge, jury, and prosecutor—understand postpartum psychiatric ill-ness? Or do they think they understand based on "conventional wis-dom" that is in fact out of touch with the realities of this illness? Does the prosecutor have political ambitions that will bias his judgment?

Was she lucky enough to have done things that would persuade a jury she was mentally ill and not to have done things that would challenge a jury's ability to understand?

In cases involving a homicide, the difference between probation and the death penalty may be a matter of *luck*. In other cases, *luck* may determine whether a woman is permitted custody of her children or is imprisoned for child endangerment. If, because of her illness, she abandoned her family, luck may determine whether she regains any parental rights. Often luck plays such a large part that it influences the outcome of the case much more than anything about the woman herself.

One way to help these women is to have attorneys in each jurisdiction who are willing to take these cases and are knowledgable about this illness. For many women this could literally make the difference between life and death.

Although judicial recognition of this illness could also greatly relieve the uncertainty and injustice these women face, on a national level, legislation of such recognition is unlikely anytime soon. Of course the best possible change would be that we would have medical procedures that would prevent these tragedies—or even this illness. To that end there is proposed federal legislation that would fund research and screening and mandate that these women are offered treatment.

It would be naïve to believe that passage of this legislation would immediately prevent all postpartum tragedies. There is much that we don't know about cause and treatment. Our health care delivery system is far from perfect. Furthermore, the nature of this illness often causes a woman to refuse treatment or attempt to fool her medical caregivers. Better medical care, de-stigmatization of mental illness, more research, and education are certain to save lives as well as pave the way for greater justice within the legal system.

PART II

Stories of Recovery

These stories were generously provided by "ordinary" women in hopes of helping others. Of course these women are not ordinary any longer in the sense that they have experienced a rare and incredibly disturbing disorder. But beyond that, these women are extraordinary for their courage, passion, and commitment to helping others, even if it means risking additional suffering. Most offered to use their real names, all face some risk of potential exposure in spite of the use of fictional names, for none of them are completely alone in knowing the details of their own story. These stories are not intended as fine literature or exquisite prose. They are simply real women's experiences with this harrowing illness.

These stories were written by women with different backgrounds, levels of education, and professional achievement. I did not make any attempt to portray this illness as one that affects any particular group of people. I requested stories through PSI, through a local newspaper, and through presentations I gave. I even included a request to spread the word that I was looking for stories in my holiday letters to family and friends.

Contributors often asked what I wanted them to include. They asked if they could talk about the birth, about their family, their past. My instruction was to include whatever *they* thought was relevant to *their* story. For that is what these are, *their* stories.

It does not seem likely that the reader will *enjoy* these stories. But I believe readers will be moved by them and will learn from them.

Chapter 5

Women Like Me, and You: Teresa's Story

It is easy now to look back on events in my life before I had children and see myself as a rather obvious candidate for postpartum depression, or even PPP (postpartum psychosis). But that was not what I thought at the time. Nor were any questions asked that would have revealed my risk. At some point during my pregnancy I may have been given a standard risk analysis form with "previous diagnosis of depression" as one of the things to check. But I was not aware of any personal or family history of depression at the time. I was aware of family history of alcoholism, eating disorders, and my own "Irish temper," but I wasn't asked about that.

Although I would sometimes say, "I'm depressed," I didn't think I had clinical depression. I thought depression meant being weepy, not being able to get out of bed, having difficulty concentrating, and so forth. Now I know that depression can look like that, but it can also mean being very angry and irritable, having very negative self-thoughts, obsessing over the negative or over past mistakes—symptoms with which I am well acquainted. (Of course most people experience anger and irritability and self-criticism—I think this is largely a matter of scale.) I would also have bouts of frenetic energy and insomnia—sometimes going for several days without sleep. But I did not think I had a "problem." I largely channeled my energy and anger and, to a large extent, learned to use it productively. Plus, like many people who have mood disorders, I could always blame the negative events in my life for my moods. So the last thing I expected was a postpartum mood disorder.

After all, I had a loving, supportive husband. We planned this baby. Although I was ambivalent about becoming pregnant, once we knew I was, I fell deeply and fiercely in love with my baby. I did not expect to have such strong feelings for a being that I could not even see or hold. I used to dismiss miscarriages, thinking, "better now than after you get attached to a baby," although I had some sympathy for the mother's disappointment. But now I realized for the first time that a miscarriage can be a tragedy. Less than two months pregnant and I already felt attached.

I had a good relationship with my parents. It had been stormy at times in the past, but there was always an awareness of love and caring. My parents lived only an hour away, so I figured I would have plenty of social support. I planned a natural birth—a couple of weeks to revel in the arrival of my new baby and then a return to my home-based professional mediation practice.

I considered myself a strong person. I knew that due to raging hormones I might get weepy and have the baby blues, but I was not really concerned about it. I even had a touch of that in my third trimester. (Or so I thought at the time—looking back I recognize it as full-blown depression.)

And I suppose I thought that severe postpartum depression was quite rare and happened to "other women"—those sorts who have major mental or situational problems already. I'm not sure if I'd ever even heard of PPP—I doubt I had. I mostly thought postpartum depression would appear as a weepy woman who would not or could not get out of bed to care for her child. I knew that some women kill their babies—I just figured those were women who did not want the child and were driven to desperate means due to extreme circumstances—an abusive relationship, pregnancy by an affair or by mistake, or being a teen mother with punitive parents.

I did not fit the picture I had of women who might end up with postpartum mood disorders—so I didn't pay much attention to that. And when I developed PPP and postpartum depression, I was taken completely by surprise.

Prior to having children I was a litigation attorney and then a professional mediator. I'd attended law school on scholarship, primarily because of scoring highly on the Law School Admissions Test (LSAT). By the time my daughter was born, I had spent over a year building an employment and business mediation practice. I was a pioneer in my field, and I loved what I did. My practice held the promise for both a substantial income and the satisfaction of doing something I believed in and felt was a contribution to our society.

My husband Drew and I had been married for almost a year when I became pregnant. We had a very good marriage. I had never really believed the "when you meet the right man, you'll know" philosophy of some of my elders. But with Drew, I knew. Our courtship and marriage was as happy a time in my life as I could remember.

My pregnancy was fairly easy with a few minor physical annoyances. From the beginning I eagerly read about every week of development. (I even bought extra books because I was too impatient to just read the ones with monthly updates.) I tried to remind myself during the first three months to not get too attached as I had a medical condition that increased my chances of miscarriage. But I knew right away I would be devastated if I lost our baby.

Drew and I went to Lamaze class (which we loved), and we even went to a birth masseuse to learn pain relief and labor-assisting techniques for natural childbirth. During the last trimester I became very annoyed with Drew for not being as involved in the pregnancy as I thought he should be. Although he did go to the classes with me, he rarely practiced with me. I felt he was more interested in doing "circus tricks" we had learned (like pushing on a certain part of my leg to make the baby move) than he was in doing the things that would bring me relief or the things we would need to do during delivery. I finally yelled at him one night, telling him he was going to have to remember these things and take the initiative as I would not be able to tell him what to do when I was in labor. During this time I had grown very angry with him for what I perceived as breaking our agreement to be responsible for this baby together.

Six days after the due date I finally went into labor. After about twelve hours of labor we asked the midwife to break my water as I was not dilating. Up until then I'd labored well. From four o'clock to midnight I labored at home. One nurse even commented that she'd never seen a woman have that much control in labor. When we broke my water I immediately went into transition. When it was time to push, the midwife asked if it was okay with us if the student midwife "caught" my daughter as she came out. I didn't care *who* did *what* so I said yes. Both the midwife and the student midwife stepped away. From nearby I heard the midwife telling me: "hold on, hold on, don't push." But finally I could not stop it and my body just pushed. I felt a huge pain. My husband was watching in the mirror and later told me that my baby's shoulders came out together and then there was a lot of blood. And I tore and tore. But I did not know that at the time.

What followed is disjointed in my memory, and I am not sure of the sequence. I remember shaking violently. My mother told me later that my shaking had terrified her. It had not scared me as I knew some women shake after delivery. I also remember my baby, Ariana, being placed on my stomach. The midwife and nurses kept telling me to put my hand on her. "Hold her, Teresa! Put your hand on her. Hold her!" I was aware of my left hand on my baby under the coverlet, but I could not speak and could not move my right hand. Finally someone took my right hand and placed it on my baby.

Then they took my baby away, and I was told I had to push out the placenta. Bummer. I thought I was done. So I pushed. The placenta came out in bits and pieces, and I kept feeling sharp pains as I passed it. Then someone began asking in an urgent tone, "Where is all the blood coming from? Where is all the blood coming from?" Now I was scared.

The midwife explained that I had a large tear and was losing blood. It was a third-degree tear, but the midwife said she was concerned about the blood loss so she offered to stitch it up. (Technically a doctor was required to repair a third-degree tear. I think it was fear of hemorrhage that prompted her to make an exception.)

On the very first stitch I screamed. And I screamed. For all I know, that screaming was only in my head—but it was also the only thought there besides fear and denial. The stitching felt exactly like what it was—a needle piercing and being pushed through my skin and muscle over and over and over and over. A nurse was gracious enough to give me her hand to hold. I remember her switching hands and then trying to give me a smaller portion of her fingers. She made some remark about feeling like I was going to break her hand, but I don't really know if she was kidding or not. At the time, I didn't care, I felt like I needed to hold that hand to hold on to my sanity. I also remember wanting to tell them to take my baby out of the room so she wouldn't hear my screams. I did not want her to be traumatized by it. I kept thinking, "No!" and "It is supposed to be DONE! Over! THIS IS ALL WRONG!"

I have thought since then that if I had been prepared for this part of it, I might have handled it better. But I fought it and denied it and resented it. Much later, I learned of a medicine that can be given post-birth to block the pain during stitching. I was so angry that I had not been given that option.

That evening the staff asked us if we wanted to leave then or if we wanted to be awakened to leave by six-thirty the next morning. The center has a 24-hour policy for uncomplicated deliveries (which all of the births there are theoretically supposed to be). We were not given adequate instructions on care of the stitched area. I've wondered if this was because it was recorded as a second-degree tear. We left the birthing center in the wee hours of the morning in a drizzling rain. I was so uncomfortable riding home, trying to lean back in the reclined seat and keep my bottom from touching it. Luckily it was less than a fifteen-minute ride. When we got home, my mother-in-law met us at the car and took Ariana. As she hurried to take Ariana out of the rain, she slipped on our very uneven bricked walkway and almost fell. That moment terrified me and haunted me for weeks.

At home I began demanding drugs for the pain. I was given a prescription pain killer but began getting hives so I had to discontinue it. Although I complained to my healthcare practitioner that I needed something stronger than Tylenol, she said that I would feel better in a day or two, just give it time.

Some time in those early days my husband and my mother-in-law left the house together to go to the drugstore. I woke up very thirsty. There was no water on my nightstand. After waiting for what seemed an eternity, I tried to reach the phone on the nightstand. I couldn't. It hurt too much. I began to cry out of fear and frustration and pain. Eventually I became terrified and panicky. By the time they came home I was angry and full of desperation. I demanded that they not leave me alone like that again. They didn't seem to understand how trapped and dependent I felt.

During this time I had mixed feelings about Ariana. I loved her and loved being with her but felt so ill and weak and frustrated. I was determined to breastfeed her but could not sit up to do it. We tried to prop me up; leaning back on a mountain of pillows in the bed, I would hold her up to my chest. That was painful for my bottom (but not as much as sitting would be) and painful for my neck and shoulders. To make matters worse, my nipples felt terribly sore and painful. When I told this to my health practitioner, I was told that all new nursing mothers complain of that, it just takes some getting used to.

Then one day a woman I had met at the one La Leche League meeting I had attended appeared at my bedside. The La Leche League is an organization that advocates for, and educates women about, breastfeeding. I don't know if Drew called her or she called him. I felt incredible relief when I saw her. She told me how to nurse Ariana while lying on my side and told me of a cream called Lansinoh that would help with my nipples. I really think I would have given up on breastfeeding if she hadn't shown up when she did

My sleep during this time was odd. I would fall asleep quickly and sleep a much deeper, blacker sleep than I have ever slept before. It seemed utterly dreamless. Then I would be awakened, usually to nurse, and I would awake startled, drenched in sweat, and feeling disoriented.

Finally, several days after Ariana was born, I became convinced that my recovery was off course. I had heard that at first you feel awful but soon every day you begin to feel better and better. I was feeling worse and worse every day. Although it was late at night (on a Saturday I think), I insisted on calling the director of the center. She met us at the center around midnight. One look told her that I had an infection. She told me she was going to swab to get a culture. I fought back tears and pleaded with her NOT to touch me THERE—not even gently. I didn't feel like I could *stand* any more pain, I couldn't cope with the pain I had.

A few days later I was taking antibiotics for the infection and beginning to feel better. My nipples were not feeling much better, but breastfeeding was much easier. I was no longer sleeping "the sleep of the dead." I was indeed beginning to feel better every day. I began to revel in my daughter. My mother-in-law, Edna, was still with us, so all I had to do was concentrate on healing and being with my daughter. One day as I was nursing and chatting with my mother-in-law, I gazed lovingly down at my perfect little cherub. I admired her soft rosy cheeks, fat and limp baby arms, and tiny perfect fingers. I felt overcome by love, and I remarked to Edna that I could not imagine how *anyone* could even *think* of hurting such a helpless, innocent creature—and not just mine, but any baby.

Little did I know how soon and how frequently I'd have those thoughts myself. The day before Edna left I was carrying Ariana past the top of the stairs when I imagined myself throwing her down the stairs. (I now know this was an OCD-type intrusive thought.) I went into the bedroom and sat down, shaking and crying. I was appalled that I could have such an awful thought. I felt like a horrible mother. It occurred to me to ask Edna to stay. But she was heading off to visit my sister-in-law who was also having her first baby. And besides, what could I give her as a reason? By all outward appearances we were beginning to manage. We were beginning to notice that my physical recovery was not proceeding as rapidly as we had hoped when I had started the medicine, but the outlook was good. And I simply could not bring myself to tell her of my awful thought or the fear it had caused in me. I was afraid if I asked her without an explanation it would look like I thought I couldn't handle motherhood on my own. Which, of course, was exactly how I felt.

I have sometimes characterized the thought I had as an "urge." When I was a teenager driving on curvy mountain roads I would sometimes imagine steering off a cliff. I would immediately fear that I might actually *do* it. The thought plus the fear made me think of these experiences as "urges." Yet I knew that I did not *want* to drive off the road. At the same time I would wonder if a part of me wanted to do it—it was the only explanation I had for why I would have such thoughts. Plus, when I was feeling suicidal as a teen, my reaction was not only fear, it was also the typical thoughts that my death would be a release, a relief. Still, it is important to understand that if I had *wanted* to go off the cliff, I could have. I didn't. I did not know for a very long time that these intrusive thoughts are characteristic of obsessive-compulsive disorder. I had other indications of this disorder as well, but I did not know it; I simply thought of myself as a "worrywart."

These intrusive thoughts about throwing my child down the stairs continued. They were so disturbing and frequent that I tried to avoid carrying her past the stairs for fear that I might not be able to restrain myself. I was too scared to sleep with her in my bed for I was certain I would roll over and suffocate her. I couldn't even sleep with her in the room for every time she made any noise I would worry something was wrong, but if she slept soundly I would be certain she had stopped breathing, so I would need to check—which inevitably would wake her up. I remember lying awake in the dark staring at her to see if her chest was moving and lying still with my eyes closed waiting to hear a little sigh, a turn, something. If it did not come soon enough I would be overcome with fear and would have to move her to see if she would awake. I was terrified of SIDS. The thought of it would haunt me at night. We finally solved this by having my husband sleep with her at night. But during the day I could not nap—or do much when she was napping for I was doubly sure that SIDS would strike then, and in my increasingly paranoid mindset I thought my husband would blame me. In my paranoia I began to become certain that my husband (who really is one of the world's greatest men and husbands) was out to get me. I thought he wanted to divorce me and take our child. Although we talked about getting help, I secretly thought he was probably sabotaging our efforts. This man, who I trust more than anyone in the world, I felt I could not trust.

I also began to resent him. I was angry that he would leave the house to go off to do work or other things. Couldn't he see how frightened I was? Couldn't he see how much I needed his help? But at the same time he began to resent me because he did not understand what was happening either. One situation that exacerbated this was an auditory hallucination I had repeatedly. I would be upstairs, and I would hear the door being unlocked, the door opening, footsteps crossing the floor, a thud like a briefcase being put on the couch, the rattling of paper. I would think it was Drew so I would call down to him and get no answer. I would grow worried that it was an intruder. (It did not occur to me to wonder WHY an intruder would bring in a briefcase and start going through papers.) I would call Drew at work and tell him to come home—there was someone in the house. He would come home to check things out, of course finding nothing. I did this over and over. He thought I was hearing squirrels on the roof and grew very annoyed that I kept calling him to come home. I grew upset that he did not respond as quickly and seemed annoyed at me for calling him (which of course fed my paranoia). He did not say to me that he thought I was hearing squirrels, and I did not tell him the details of what I was hearing. Had either of us known about auditory hallucinations, maybe we would have explored this odd, recurring problem more thoroughly.

I got to the point where I was terrified to be alone with my daughter. At one point I phoned my mom to beg her to come. She is a professor and has summers off, so I thought she would certainly come if she knew I needed her. Besides, this was her first and only grandchild, and my parents had talked repeatedly about how much they wanted a grandchild. Surely she would come for at least one night. I called and left a desperate, pleading message on the answering machine. She returned the call and left a simple message on my machine saying she had got my message but had decided not to come. I was devastated.

She had not actually heard my message but had heard through my father that I had called and wanted her to come. I see my parents as people with their own lives and careers who put a lot of emphasis on their children being independent. I remember being terribly disappointed in what I perceived to be my mother's lack of interest and involvement in my wedding. I am often disappointed now that they choose to spend such a short period of time with us when they do visit. But at the time of my psychosis, this disappointment had a very different quality. In my mind, my mother's refusal to come gave credence to my fears and paranoia. It indicated a complete abandonment, not only by her but by everyone.

Later, when I learned that my father conveyed the message, it made sense to me that my mom would not come. I believe my father saw me as an unreasonable, highly emotional, oversensitive person. Therefore what seemed to be pleading and desperation to me struck him as overreacting. This is not all his fault. I have often been loud and volatile, especially where my father is concerned. In other words, this probably seemed like NORMAL behavior to him. It did not occur to him or to me that my past behavior might be related to a mood disorder as well.

It is hard to give a complete picture of my postpartum period. Much of it is fuzzy now. I can think of no better word than desperate. Deeply, darkly desperate. Yet I know that I smiled and joked. I changed diapers and cooed at my baby. I did dishes and returned phone calls. I don't really remember doing that, but I must have. If I hadn't, surely someone would have noticed something seriously wrong.

But I hid it. No one knew that I could not really follow a television program. I liked having the TV on. When I would hear things that I recognized as auditory hallucinations I would blame them on the TV even when I *knew* they were not coming from the TV. I also could not read. The letters would be readable for a few words or so, but then they began to look like hieroglyphs—I could not read them; no matter how hard I tried, I could not make sense of them. That was particularly scary because I had never heard of such a thing before.

I would hear people talking and whispering. I would hear voices coming from the other rooms upstairs when I knew nobody was there. I even heard them coming from a "room" that was not even there—so I *knew* nobody was *there*. At the same time I worried that these people were plotting against me and laughing at me.

The worst part of my experience was a solitary visual hallucination. When I first prepared to share my story I found myself pouring out something I'd not intended to share. This was the single worst incident of my postpartum experience. I frequently describe it as the worst experience of my life. Putting this in perspective: I've experienced rape, cancer, and rejection by family. Here is the retelling as I experienced it.

I am lying on the bed that I share with my husband, Drew. Our newborn daughter, Ariana, is lying next to me. She has just finished nursing and is now sleeping peacefully. I'm not thinking anything in particular—or hearing anything—or feeling anything. I look down and see a pair of scissors—shiny, silver, metal scissors with an orange handle—in my right hand. I take the scissors, and I place the sharp point at the hollow of her neck. I push the point of the scissors in and then quickly cut, slicing from her neck down to her pubis. Blood flows. Suddenly horrified, I quickly look away. I cannot bear to look at her. I wipe off the scissors on the sheet. I get up, still averting my gaze from her. I think, "I cannot believe I have imagined such a terrible thing." (Yet in spite of telling myself that I imagined it, I cannot look at her.) *I go about the room gathering up any sharp object I can find, still averting my gaze from my daughter. I take these objects down the hall to my home office. Once there, I gather up all the sharp objects I can find there. I go to a closet, open the door, place the sharp objects far in the back of the top shelf. I figure I will have to think twice before I get those objects and that perhaps in doing that I won't actually act upon an impulse to hurt my child with them. Then I think maybe I should throw myself and her down the stairs together. The likelihood is that she would die and I would not, even if I were injured. A sort of peaceful feeling that life could go back to the way it was—that my husband would love me again—that we would be free—that I would be free—comes across my mind. At the same time I know this is not true. I feel a fierce protective love for my daughter. I don't want to kill her. But I think maybe sometimes I do—after all, I have these bad thoughts. I've wanted to tell my husband about this, but I'm afraid he's looking for a reason to leave me. I'm afraid if I tell him he will have me locked up and will leave with the baby. Or worse yet, if I tell someone, and I'm not believed, or I'm just told to get over it or something—if I seek treatment but do not get it, or the treatment does not work, and I kill my child—I could be prosecuted for first degree murder! I could get the death penalty! I wish I were in England where the most I could get for infanticide is manslaughter. If I were in England, I could tell someone what I am feeling and thinking. I slowly go back toward the bedroom. I am trembling at the horrid thought that I had. I cross the threshold into the bedroom. I see my baby lying there on the bed, the blood covering the sheets, dripping on the floor. I am absolutely horrified that I have killed my child. This innocent, helpless child whom I love! I stand there for a moment staring—too shocked to scream. Or maybe I do scream and no one hears—I can't be sure. I feel like my life is over. I want my life to be over. I don't want my life to be over.*

I don't know how long I stood there. Was it seconds, minutes, an hour? I don't know when I realized that she was okay. I don't know if I blinked, looked away, if there was some merge in my vision. All I know is that one moment I was looking at my dead child, lying on the bed, exposed. Then there was blackness. Then I was looking at my child safely and peacefully sleeping on the bed.

It took me a year and a half to share that story with my husband. Although this was the worst episode of my postpartum depression, it was also the shortest. I don't know how long I was paranoid, hearing voices, unable to read, and so on. But eventually those symptoms faded, and I was left simply deeply depressed.

There are many things about my experience that are difficult to explain. For example, I can honestly tell you that I never felt "suicidal." I *did* have that moment of feeling like I wanted my life to be over. But I did not want to kill myself; I did not want to be dead. It was a thought and a feeling, not a desire.

Also, it is hard to fully explain the difference between this hallucination and the other thoughts I had. What I *can* say is that experientially they were *very* different. The thoughts about throwing my daughter down the stairs occurred as mental images. They were in the "mind's eye," so to speak. I had no doubt they were thoughts. When I talk of them now, I can talk very matter-of-factly about them. These thoughts would occur in my mind fully formed—not like a still photo—but like a concept fully formed. Like a memory of something. There is no mystery about what is going to happen.

The hallucination felt like it was actually happening. It did not occur to me as a thought. When I got up from the bed I *told* myself it was a terrible thought, and that was what I wanted to believe. But I was also afraid to look at my daughter. It is as if on one level I was afraid I had done it, and on another level I did not think I could do something like that, so I was reassuring myself that it was just a thought. Even then I knew it was very different from the other disturbing thoughts I'd been having. But I wanted to believe it was a thought *just like those other thoughts* even though I knew the experience was *not* the same.

When I recount this story to others, I cry. It is still so emotional because I remember it the way you would remember something that was real, even though I know it was not. (And it is terrifying to think what might have been.) To this day, I don't know at what point I picked up the scissors. I know I had them in my hand to put in the closet but whether I had them in my hand when I had the hallucination, I don't know. I still do not know whether the action of wiping the scissor blades on the sheets was something I did or something I imagined.

If I *had* killed my daughter, and I was asked if I had "wanted" to kill her, I probably would have said "yes." *Not* because I wanted to kill her. I never *wanted* to kill her, I never *wanted* her dead. But I felt such guilt over the thoughts I had, and I was so used to thinking of other "urges" or intrusive thoughts as a reflection of desire, that I probably would have said "yes." I had no other way of understanding it. I've communicated with and read about a number of women who had PPP and several who committed infanticide. I have yet to know of any who *wanted* to kill their child or *wanted* their child dead.

Also, even though I feared I killed my daughter, even though I hid sharp implements to protect her from *me*, I also did not believe that *I* could or would ever hurt my child. I know myself. I know I strive to be and am considered by others to be a good and loving person, a good and loving mother. I know it is not in my nature to do such a thing. It isn't as if I've never done bad or hurtful things. I still feel guilty for stealing a salt shaker from a Wendy's when I was in college. I still feel guilty for making a cruel comment about one of my class-mates in law school. But I am not the kind of person who would physi-cally harm a child. What I did not know was that who *I am* as a moral being has nothing to do with what happened or might have happened.

When I recently interviewed Dr. Margaret Spinelli, an eminent authority in this field, she told me of having to warn families that this "gentle and nice" mother may be a threat to her child. "This has nothing to do with her [the woman]," Spinelli explained, "This is the illness." She paused, "Or as we say [in the field], it's chemistry not character."[1]

I realize much of this is difficult to understand. Much of it is diffi-cult to explain. That is one of the reasons I wanted to do this book. I feel that in order to fight the stigma that this illness faces, it is impor-tant for people to know what it is like to experience this strange and sometimes tragic illness.

When I recovered from the psychosis, I sunk into a deep, severe depression. I did not know it at the time and did not get help. I've since learned this is a common transition for women with PPP.

I spent a lot of time fretting that I was not bonding with my daugh-ter. I was consumed with the feeling that I had made a giant mistake, and I simply was not cut out to be a mother. I even thought about put-ting my daughter up for adoption (although just the *thought* broke my heart—even today, just *remembering* that makes me cry) but knew my husband would not consider it. Even as I was having these thoughts, he started talking about having another child. I was so angry at him for that, but did not say anything. Couldn't he see how miserable I was—how desperate—how inadequate? But I could not tell him all that or I would have to tell him about all the terrible thoughts I had experi-enced. And I still was not at a place where I could see my condition clearly. So the paranoia of the past did not occur to me as paranoia but as possible reality.

Normally I am not a passive person. But when my husband pushed for a second child, I went along with it. I had nothing in me to resist his request. We did conceive a second time. I had many difficulties with this pregnancy. I was very nauseous, extremely tired all the time—the opposite of my first pregnancy. I was convinced something was wrong. I thought that maybe I was pregnant with twins, but after several tests and reassurances that it was a singleton, I gradually came to accept that it was just one child—but feared that there was some-thing terribly wrong with him or her.

Finally, when I was five-and-a-half months along, we had our first routine sonogram. In a matter of moments, we were told that we were expecting twin girls and that they were monoamniotic. Monoamniotic twins share one amniotic sac and have very high mortality and morbidity rates. We were immediately counseled on the possibility of "selective reduction," but said, "No!" I spent the next month in an intense state of worry. The more I learned about monoamniotics, the more bad news I discovered. I also learned that depression is more prevalent in mothers of multiples, and child abuse is higher in families of multiples.

Just before I started bedrest I changed doctors and discovered that my twins were not monoamniotic. It was a *huge* relief, but I was still worried about possible postpartum depression.

While on bedrest I started spending time on the Internet. In a chat room one day someone asked about postpartum depression and hallucinations. I wrote that I had postpartum depression and hallucinations. Someone wrote to me and said she was a nurse and what I was describing was "PPP." I became more fearful of my upcoming postpartum period and decided I had to share some of my story with my family so they could guard in case it happened again.

The first person I told was my sister-in-law. She patiently sat on the phone with me (long distance) while I sobbed for over thirty minutes before I could even *begin* to tell my story. At the time I would have laughed out loud in rueful disbelief if someone had suggested that one day I would share my story in a book. I told my family that if I acted strange at all or said anything strange, or seemed agitated, to get me to a doctor right away.

And then the strangest thing happened, the twins were born, and I was fine. I thought "Oh, THIS is what it is supposed to feel like!" A week after they were born I had to persuade my family that it was okay to leave the three children with me for a few hours alone. But I was not the least bit nervous—I *knew* I was perfectly fine—physically and mentally.

The PPP was, as far as I was concerned, in the past and buried. I did not intend to ever speak of it again. Then Andrea Yates drowned her five children in a bathtub in Texas. The more I heard about her the more I was convinced that this woman must have had PPP. I knew I needed to share my story with others.

I went through a lot of emotional turmoil over having had PPP (what I now call post-recovery recovery). I searched for reasons *why* this would happen to me. I grieved the lost quality time with my daughter. I had to learn to trust myself again. I grappled with fear of a recurrence. I processed the anger I had over not being diagnosed and treated. I'd like to say I got over my fear of stigma. But that would not be true; I still sometimes get concerned about what people will think of me—a woman who had psychosis. A woman who has been mentally ill!

Ironically, I'm probably more mentally *well* now than ever before in my life! My father once asked, "What is your first memory of a symptom you'd associate with bipolar?" I think it was second grade. It was a feeling of a big grey-black cloud of rage and an accompanying thought that I needed to control it and hide it.

I still have obsessive-compulsive thoughts occasionally. Usually my old standby of having a house fire at night and feeling the need to check the smoke alarms. But they are not a problem; I know how to manage them. And I believe that I probably have "soft bipolar" or "bipolar II." But it too is not an issue; I take Bupropion and that seems to manage it well.

There is so much I'd like to see change. I believe if I'd had a thorough history taken, if I'd been examined regarding my mood postpartum, if I'd had knowledgeable medical providers and caregivers, things would have been different. It also hurts me to know that so many in my own profession, law, are ignorant of the realities of mental illness and how greatly that contributes to suffering and injustice.

I'm still learning. I recently attended a conference where some presenters talked about looking at a woman's reproductive history, particularly reproductive traumas, as predictors for postpartum mood complications. When I wrote my list, I forgot to put "rape" on it! It is amazing how much trauma we allow people to suffer without aid. I had been told in my late teens and early twenties that I almost certainly could not have children due to my history of ovarian cysts. (Ironically this started a year after the rape.) It was emotionally traumatic. But amazingly, those doctors never recommended that I talk to someone about how I *felt* about that!

It is absurd that it is not *routine* to evaluate postpartum women for mood disorders, particularly those who had experienced trauma or have complications. When I was wheeled into the birthing center (because it was too painful to walk) for a postpartum checkup, I was asked "How are you doing?" I completely broke down, crying and sobbing and saying I could not handle it. I was then promptly wheeled into an examination room—for a physical exam. There was no other mention of my emotional state. Perhaps they thought that because I had a good reason to be upset, they did not have to be concerned with it. That seems to be prevalent in our culture—we don't need to be concerned about depression or anger if there is a good reason for it. In fact, I often used that rationale on myself when I had "bad days" (which could last weeks). I did not think I had a mood disorder; I had plenty of reasons to be angry and upset.

Even in the postpartum period, too often we expect the ill person to be the one to seek help. That becomes complicated when the person is mentally ill in a society that stigmatizes mental illness. For those with PPP this is particularly difficult. The woman may be unaware or uneducated about the illness, available resources, or the risks involved; plus she is probably paranoid and may not realize what she is experiencing is not real. We cannot place the burden of self-diagnosis on these mothers. We must do a better job of risk assessment through thorough histories, prevention, diagnosis, and treatment. We must educate the public and professionals.

Too often women do not tell others what they are suffering. I didn't. Like many women, on one hand I feared that I would not be believed; on the other hand I feared the stigma of mental illness. So instead, I hid it—and in doing so I spent a painful two years barely surviving and not being the mother that my daughter deserves, or that I deserve.

I am now happy and enjoy my three lovely daughters. Yet I still have to chuckle when someone comments, "You are such a natural mother, you make it look so effortless." I don't feel that way, but compared to how I felt when I was ill—when every *moment* was a struggle—it comes close.

Chapter 6

After the Manic "Super Mom" Period: Laura's Story

It seems overwhelming to write about the events that took place after the birth of my son. However, I am compelled to share this story because it is a story of hope. My biggest desire is to be a source of hope for those women who cannot see the light at the end of the tunnel. I hope that the real-life story that is told in the following pages will be used to help suffering mothers and their confused and scared families. Before I go into the details of my postpartum experience, I would like to share a little bit about my life surrounding these events. I believe strongly that the stress that was occurring in my life led to the postpartum problems that I experienced. I was married to Thomas, a "recovering" drug addict who was far from recovery. We discovered that we were pregnant (our first child) in January of 1999. Throughout my entire pregnancy, I lived the co-dependent lifestyle that usually goes along with being married to an addict. I was heavily stressed with the pressures of living with an addict, and I felt overwhelmed with the thought of bringing a new baby into this world under such unstable conditions. Thomas (my now ex-husband) remained on the roller-coaster ride of addiction throughout our two-and-a-half year marriage.

Our son, Isaac, was born in September, 1999. My labor was amazingly easy and everything (as far as Isaac went) was going smoothly during those first two weeks home from the hospital. I was breastfeeding, and we were able to get Isaac onto a good schedule within the first couple of days. However, I was not sleeping at all. I was extremely talkative and excited, and I did everything for the baby. I was "super mom," as some would call it. We later learned that all of the symptoms that I was experiencing were part of a manic episode. My husband and I were living with my parents, and so I had plenty of people to notice how strange I was acting.

I had become extremely spiritual, singing and praying constantly as I walked through the house and cared for Isaac. I felt more "one" with God than I had ever felt in my life. Everything that I did was very meticulous. It took me at least an hour to get all of Isaac's stuff together for a simple outing to the doctor or to church. I can remember going to get reprints of some snapshots we had taken of Isaac, and I was very obsessive about the whole situation. I still have a multitude of pictures from that time period. My family reports that I talked excessively and would not be still. I was constantly thinking about what I needed to do next. Every time I tried to sleep, I thought of something that I would rather do with the short amount of time that I had before the next feeding. I felt like every second of my time had to be used wisely. All of this behavior lasted for two weeks, until I snapped.

My husband and I had just taken Isaac to the doctor for his two-week appointment, and we were heading home. I was driving, and Thomas was in the passenger seat. I started singing a song, and Thomas began to get frustrated with me. He told me that I was going to wake the baby up, and I instantly turned on him. In my mind, he was being controlled by evil spirits, and that is why he didn't want me to sing. So, I pulled the car over into a parking lot and began trying to cast these spirits out in the name of Jesus. Thomas became very scared and quickly picked up our cell phone to call my parents. By this time we had both gotten out of the car, and Thomas was trying to get away from me as he called my parents.

Soon, an ambulance arrived, and I was forced to go to the hospital. In my mind, I was really okay, and all that I could think about was the fact that my baby would be hungry soon. I was taken into the emergency room, and my mom waited with me for the doctor. I can remember the anger that I felt toward my mom as she began telling the doctor about what little sleep I had been getting. I finally told my mom to leave and would not allow her to see me for the entire first week. They admitted me into a mental hospital.

I can remember trying to talk to the nurses when I first got there, in attempts to make them believe that I really wasn't crazy. I believed that everything I was dealing with was a result of spiritual warfare. I would go into the bathroom and pray out loud, trying to fight the evil that I felt was so present. Upon being admitted, I began fighting and trying to get away. The nurses had to gather around me and force me to the floor in order to inject me with Haldol. All of these memories are extremely vivid in my mind. It was a complete nightmare. It took them a few days to get me "down" from my manic high. But after they got me down, I began what my family began calling "the Haldol shuffle." I was very drugged and sluggish. The doctors told us that I needed to be in this "zombie" state in order for my brain to heal. They explained that I had experienced postpartum psychosis, which is characterized by a manic episode followed by severe depression. It was like having one episode of bipolar disorder.

After two weeks, I was discharged and sent home. Looking back, my family reflects on how little information they were given upon my discharge. They felt extremely helpless and alone as they began caring for me. There was no support offered from the medical community, but, thankfully, we were blessed with wonderful friends and neighbors who tried their best to support us. I am not going to try to go into what my family was dealing with, because it is hard enough to describe what was happening inside of me. I remained in the "zombie" state once I returned home.

Upon my release from the hospital, my case was turned over to a local outpatient mental health facility. I was supposed to go to appointments there, in order to keep my medication regulated. The care that I received at this place was very disappointing. The time period is very cloudy for me because of the high dosage of Haldol that I was receiving. But, I remember my husband and I asking the doctor if he could lower my dosage of Haldol because I was in such a "zombie" state. He immediately agreed to do so, and my dose was cut in half. As I remember, that was the one and only time I went for an appointment there. Within a few days of reducing my dosage, a strange thing happened; I slipped into a deep, vegetative depression. I guess when I was on the full dosage of Haldol, I was too out of it to be depressed.

Keep in mind, that during this entire time following my manic episode, I was unable to care for Isaac. He had been put on formula immediately, and unfortunately developed colic. So, my family was dealing with me and a crying baby at the same time. I felt like I was in hell.

The doctors told my family to keep me on a schedule. So, my mom would come and wake me up every morning around eight o'clock, and I would go upstairs to waste my day away on the couch. I had no desire to eat, and I couldn't sleep unless I took sleeping pills. Throughout the entire day, I laid on the couch watching the clock. My mom or my husband took care of the baby, and they would try to get me to do something every now and then. I can remember my mom putting my baby beside me on the couch, and within one minute, I was ready for her to come and get him.

My son spent a lot of time in his swing the first couple of months, and I would become extremely anxious if I was left in the room by myself with him. If my husband went out onto the porch to smoke a cigarette, I felt tense until he returned. I felt incapable of dealing with anything. It felt like a chore to get up and take a shower or brush my teeth. My arms literally ached when I washed my hair. I was very weak, and my brain felt like it was barely functioning. As a result, my appearance was not normal. I didn't put on my makeup or fix my hair like normal, because my mind wasn't functioning properly. I literally lay on the couch all day, until I could take my medication at 8:00 P.M. and go to bed.

I can remember my sixteen-year-old sister leaving to go somewhere early in the day with her boyfriend, and me still being in the same place when they returned. This went on for about one month after my first hospitalization, and we finally called my psychiatrist in desperation. He informed us that the fastest way to get me out of the vegetative depression would be electroconvulsive therapy. At that point, we were willing to try anything that looked hopeful. So, I was re-admitted to the mental hospital, and electroconvulsive therapy began. I was given a total of six treatments over a two-week time period. The treatments made me very confused—so that time period is a big blur.

I was released from the hospital right before Christmas. My family was not prepared to see me in such a confused state. It was as if I had to re-learn how to do things that should have come naturally. My brain was so sluggish that I couldn't even help bake cookies without being given step-by-step instructions. It took me about two weeks to recuperate, and at that point, I was able to care for my baby and function enough to take a shower and drive a car. But, contrary to what we expected, I was nowhere near myself. I was still depressed, and from January until March I stayed inside my house all day while I cared for my baby. I would put him in his swing and pray that he would stay asleep so that I wouldn't have to interact with him. My mom was very worried about me and called me regularly throughout the day while she was at work. I remember trying to motivate myself to clean the house and take Isaac for a walk in his stroller. I knew that these things would be good for me, but I was unable to make myself do what I needed to do. My Mom began searching for a doctor who could help me, and that is when she discovered the North Carolina Depression After Delivery (DAD) group. She was able to talk to mothers who had been through similar situations, and they referred her to Dr. Pederson at UNC-Chapel Hill. She was able to make an appointment for me, and I was first seen by Dr. Pederson in March. It had been five and a half months since my first hospitalization, and I was desperate for help.

Dr. Pederson talked to me and found out the current medications that I was taking. He immediately put me on a thyroid medication and began weaning me off of the Paxil that I was taking. Within three or four days, I was beginning to take an interest in conversations around me. I was showing emotions, and my family was amazed. After weaning me off of the Paxil, I was put on Wellbutrin (Bupropion) and continued taking Lithium. I was completely back to my normal self within one month of seeing Dr. Pederson for the first time.

I have not had any relapses since recovering, and at the present time I am a senior at Carolina University. I have faced some enormous struggles since my recovery, and have not slipped back into depression. My family and I remain amazed at what has happened in my life, and I want to offer hope to those families who are caught in the middle of this sickness. I recovered in March of 2000 and remained stable throughout a year of living with a drug addict. In February of 2001, my ex-husband and I separated due to his continued drug abuse, and by August of 2001 I had moved two hours away from my family with my two-year-old to attend college. Since going back to school, I have maintained a 3.4 average in the midst of dealing with the termination of my ex-husband's parental rights, and a divorce. I remained on my medication until October of 2001, and, at that point, I began weaning myself off, under my doctor's supervision.

I am majoring in psychology, and it has been amazing to learn about postpartum psychosis in my classes, as well as other disorders. What started out as a complete nightmare has turned into something amazing. I am thankful for the experience that I encountered because I have knowledge of what it is like to have a mental disorder. I was able to realize what I want to do with my life as a result of my experience. I have a burning desire to reach out to women who are experiencing postpartum problems. And, I have great compassion for those people who are suffering from mental disorders. I am so thankful for the inside view that I have as a result of the suffering that I endured. I am in no way trying to brag about how wonderful I am doing now. I want people to realize that my family felt just as hopeless as many others do now. My family had to come to terms with the fact that I might never be the same again. I don't want anyone to feel they have to settle for that. There is hope, and I pray that others will find out where to get the help that so many desperately need. Some women never return to their "normal" selves after the birth of their children. It is such a sad fact, and I want awareness to be raised so that people don't settle for less than what they deserve.

Chapter 7

A Story of Recovery in Five Parts: Eva's Story

PART I

My name is Eva. I am the mother of two beautiful boys. I have survived postpartum depression and psychosis, and this is my story. I dedicate this story to my sons, Peter and Thomas.

Before I had my son, Peter, I was diagnosed with clinical depression while trying to recover from alcohol and drug addiction. Depression also ran in my family. My mother has since died from a drug overdose, and my father is still a drug addict. My grandfather was also an alcoholic. I was adopted by my grandparents and raised by my aunt, whom I have called "mom" since I was small. No one told me I was already at risk for postpartum depression.

I took no antidepressants during my pregnancy; I wish I had. They weren't proven to be completely harmless while pregnant or breastfeeding. No one offered me the option anyway.

My boyfriend, Henry, and I were not married at the time. I was twenty-four years old, and he was just twenty-one. The two of us had practically just met. We lived in the basement of his parents' home throughout my pregnancy and for two years after Peter was born. The two-room suite was just enough space for the three of us. We always had enough privacy.

After I gave birth (a couple days after), I noticed my mood having extreme highs or extreme lows. The highs were happy times or what I thought a new mother should be feeling. The lows were debilitating. I felt so overwhelmed by this small six-pound life that required every ounce of energy I had. I wasn't sleeping but a couple of hours each night. The baby demanded my utmost attention twenty-four hours a day. Even if I did sleep, I did it with one eye open. Every single night

I called the twenty-four-hour baby care phone number on the brochure given to me in the hospital, titled "Getting Through The First 4 Weeks." If I wasn't calling about the baby, I was calling about me. I would sob on the telephone, "My episiotomy hurts, it must be infected," or "I'm having trouble breastfeeding." Little did I know that my lack of enthusiasm caused Peter to sense that I just wasn't into this maternal part of a newborn's life. I really wanted to breastfeed for at least six months, but I felt like a complete stranger was groping me. I didn't feel that I deserved the wonderful experience that so many mothers spoke of. I'd cry and tell these professionals on the phone that I was so overwhelmed. They summed it up to be a bad case of the baby blues. I had heard of this and thought they were right. After all, my hormones had just had a complete overhaul. But why did I feel like at any minute my world was going to come crashing down?

When Peter was ten weeks old, friends of ours lost their baby to SIDS (Sudden Infant Death Syndrome). This event sent me spiraling downward. "What if it were Peter?" "Why wasn't it Peter?"

I had terrible obsessive thoughts. My mind would hold on to them like Velcro and not be able to let go. I remember driving across a snow-covered country road and thinking, "What if I just dropped him off in this field and left him there to freeze to death?" Or I'd be doing laundry and think, "What if I just tossed my baby in the clothes dryer?" It was amazing what my mind could come up with. I could invent a harmful object from just about anything. The thoughts were like little demons creeping into my room each and every night, depriving my sleep-starved, emotionally unstable body. They were haunting. I started to hallucinate. All of the appliances now had jaws. They told me I was the devil, and I eventually started believing what they were telling me.

I was also terrified of spiders, but there was a frequent creepy crawler on my bedroom ceiling that eventually became my friend, my ear, and my confidant. This little eight-legged creature understood what I was going through. I would babble and talk nonsense. I didn't know it was wrong and couldn't grab onto it long enough to make it stop. I had lost touch with reality. Hours would go by feeling like minutes.

Henry worked only steps away, but I longed for him to arrive home. I hated being alone with these demons in my head. I hated being alone with the baby. I was so afraid I would hurt him. The urge was overwhelming. By now, I felt I had no control over anything—myself, my baby—I even started to doubt my relationship with Henry. I would compulsively clean and try to run a house that wasn't even mine. Henry supported me no matter what I did or felt but I kept asking myself, "How can he love me when all I can think about is ways I could harm our beautiful newborn?" He knew when I was most bothered by these visions by the way I would start cleaning, straightening, and organizing everyone else's things. I was terrified of what someone would think had they been a fly on the wall.

Today, my husband tells me he knew something was starting to get out of hand, but he couldn't tell anyone what was happening. I don't think he could put it into words without other family members thinking that he too was crazy. He tells me he was mostly scared of me harming myself. He knew I loved Peter too much to hurt him. If I only were convinced of that at the time, maybe I would have recovered sooner. If I told anyone, like a doctor, I was afraid he or she would take my baby away from me. This was certainly not a healthy way to commence motherhood.

I thought I was going crazy. But my thoughts were real. They were very real. They were repetitive and strong. Nothing I did could make them go away. I would think my way into hysterics. Guilt would then haunt me as if I really committed this monstrous act. I had a panic attack one time, and I will never forget it. I was sitting in the movie theatre seeing *Titanic*. At the end, when the majority of the ship's passengers were frozen in the water, the movie showed a mother holding her baby, the same age as Peter, both of them dead. I was with Henry and two of my girlfriends. I ran out of the theatre not able to breathe, sobbing uncontrollably. I took the fastest way to the outside and sat down against the building with my head buried in my knees. I was so hysterical—I had sat in a mud puddle and didn't even know it. With snot and tears running down my face, I realized that I wasn't surprised that this was how I reacted to that scene in the movie. Henry followed me out and kneeled down beside me. He held me for about five minutes until I calmed down. We both knew it was time I got some help. I promised to call a doctor the next day.

Peter was about four months old by this time. I had only confided in my husband and a couple of friends. I thought anything would be better than this insanity. I wished I were dead.

A therapist told me I had postpartum depression and needed to be put on medication. I instantly agreed, for I would have done anything to get better. Sometimes, I thought it would never get better. I thought there was not hope for strange women like myself. I felt so incredibly alone. This was not how a new mother was supposed to feel. People were criticizing me because I was supposed to be happy. But I was not. I was more sad and depressed than I had ever been in my life. Asking a new mother why help was not gotten sooner totally underestimates the shame that accompanies this illness. I was so utterly ashamed of myself—I wanted to die.

Finally, after a year of trying a host of antidepressants, I finally found one that targeted the obsessive-compulsive disorder along with the depression. It's called Luvox, and it saved my life. I recall the first time I spoke with another woman who had the same kind of thoughts I did. I remember thinking, "Thank you God for not letting me be the only one." I spoke with that woman on the telephone a lot. We stuck around after the support group meetings and gabbed. We were both stable enough to talk of things other than thoughts of putting our children into microwave ovens. The new me was starting to emerge.

Today Peter is almost five years old, and I am twenty-nine. I have been married to my wonderful husband, Henry, for five years. Today, the past is one big blurred memory. I remember moments I am supposed to remember like Peter's first step, tooth, and so on—but nothing else. I think this is how it is supposed to be. Henry has been a solid column for me to lean up against when I felt I was no longer able to stay standing. I have a great support system, which is vital for me to stay well. I wasn't sure I would get postpartum depression after having another baby. I knew I was at great risk for it though. Women everywhere need to be aware of postpartum depression and if they, themselves, are at risk for it. I want mothers who have or may have postpartum depression to know that there is hope. You can get help. It does get better. But most importantly, you are not alone.

PART II

In the summer of 2001, four or five women ended their lives due to postpartum depression and psychosis. Andrea Yates was the most famed story about the disease. I felt something had to be done. Women had to speak out. I called the local newspaper, and a reporter came out to my home and interviewed me about my past experience with postpartum depression. It made it in the local paper, and she told me of a woman from the same county I was from who had been incarcerated for killing her two children before trying to kill herself. She was charged with infanticide and given a life sentence. She had been in jail for sixteen years. Her lawyers were getting together a clemency petition to try for her release. I phoned her lawyer and then began talking to this woman through letters. I attended conversation salons at her lawyer's home to learn what this project would entail. It lasted five months, and the petition finally went to the governor. Unfortunately, her petition was denied.

While the hearing was taking place, I heard they were looking for people for *The Oprah Winfrey Show* to share their stories about the illness. I emailed the show and later received an invitation to attend the taping and sit in the front row. Oprah briefly (on the air) asked me about my experience. She didn't know much about the illness, and many people were disappointed in how the show turned out. But at least the illness was starting to get publicity. I fell apart immediately after the show. I knew my medication needed to be adjusted, and that

I was falling slowly into depression again. It was November and the holidays were approaching, and my moods always fell during the holidays. My mother moved in with us to help out because, with the depression, the holidays proved to be too much. But I made it through and everyone was happy.

PART III

I went to my best friend's house the day she found out she was pregnant. I told her my period was late. She had another pregnancy test, as two came in the box. I took the test, and I wasn't too surprised it came up positive. I narrowed the time of conception down to Christmas Eve. It wasn't the most ideal time for my husband and I to have another baby, but there was something special about Liz and I being pregnant together. Her first child was the baby that died of SIDS when Peter was a newborn. We both thought it was more than irony that we were about to embark on this journey together, while neither of us was really ready and both apparently conceiving while on some type of birth control. When I came home and told my husband, he didn't believe me. I had to tell him twice. He thought the same way I did. It was what we both wanted, but it was just not the ideal time. He too thought it was neat that Liz and I were about to do it together again.

I immediately started to feel the shift of the hormones and became a little depressed. I started attending the support group for mothers with postpartum depression. I went to every Wednesday afternoon meeting, getting more pregnant as time went on. All the other women there already had their children, of course, and all had significant signs of postpartum depression. I could relate to a lot of their stories from when I had it the first time. The whole time I was pregnant, I was the only pregnant one in the meeting. I was also seeing a psychiatrist and was put on medication safe for pregnancy. I was taking Paxil and Ativan for anxiety, and Ambien for sleep. My obstetrician was aware of the meds and prepared for what could happen immediately after childbirth. Narcan, a drug used to reverse the side effects of narcotics, would be given so the baby didn't come out asleep. The anxiety from all the medication problems was heavy on my shoulders, and I often talked about it in the meetings. I was gaining so much weight, which was making me more depressed. Sex used to be great because of the hormones during pregnancy, but now I was barely interested. I mean, we hardly had it while I was pregnant. I was so huge and felt so unattractive. I started having obsessive thoughts about throwing myself off balconies or over bridges or in front of cars. Then I started getting migraine headaches that eventually were unbearable. My doctor said "hang in there"—sometimes headaches come with pregnancy. So in other words—live with it.

Around my fifth month of pregnancy, my skin all over my body started to itch. It itched so badly, I developed bruises where my fingernails would try to embed into my body. I broke blood vessels where the bruises would be. I would itch myself into hysteria and begin to cry and scream because I just couldn't take it anymore. My mother lived with us shortly before I was pregnant the second time and witnessed the whole pregnancy and tried to help where she could but felt helpless at the same time. I was told by a dermatologist that the itching was due to an elevated liver enzyme that was excreted into the skin, called bile salts. This in turn causes the skin to itch as the skin sweats. It was unbearable. I had this itching during my first pregnancy as well, and it was just as severe with this pregnancy, so I knew it would not go away until delivery. All of these events were precursors to the level of depression I had following this pregnancy.

I had a migraine one day and the doctor decided to admit me into the hospital to try and control the pain. It was still three to four weeks until my due date. She kept me overnight and gave me morphine with still no relief. The next morning my husband came in to visit, and the doctor came as well. We discussed it, and she decided to induce labor because my headache was still quite severe.

They moved me into a labor room (a very nice room) and started me on the IV drug Pitocin to make the contractions stronger. At about 6:00 P.M. I started asking for something for pain and that didn't last long. Pretty soon it was decided to give me an epidural. I had back surgery in the past, and I wasn't sure if an epidural would be effective or not. The plates and screws were in the same space that the epidural needle would go. The anesthesiologist explained to me that it might not control the pain as I had hoped, but he would give it his best shot. After he was done inserting the epidural, I felt this extremely painful sensation—like I had to push. The anesthesiologist started calling for the nurse and they barely called the doctor in time as all of a sudden I was fully dilated and ready to push the baby out. Ten minutes later, Thomas Theodore was born, and I felt every bit of it. This traumatic birth experience also affected the outcome of the postpartum period of depression.

We stayed in the hospital for a few days as mom and baby were both very healthy. When we came home, my mood immediately shifted. I cried as I stepped in the door. I knew that the first few days were a shift in hormones and a dramatic shift at that. So I tried to hang in there for the first week. But I felt like I had been hit over the head with a bat. When I finally did get to see my doctor, he confirmed what I knew was going on: another bout of postpartum depression. Once again it started with those terrible thoughts. I cried a lot and often got frustrated. I was attending a support group still and seeing my psychiatrist and thought "time will help me to get through this," of course with the help of medications, which were slightly adjusted after the birth of Thomas.

After he was about a month old, I attended a walk put on by a woman whose daughter, Melanie Stokes, jumped to her death the summer before as a result of postpartum psychosis. I felt foggy during and after the walk. I came home having hallucinations and delusions. I have been told that I was speaking to those other deceased women who passed at the hands of postpartum depression and psychosis. I knew I was acting sick and that speaking to a dead woman was irrational, but I could hear these voices and they felt so very real to me.

I was admitted into Good Samaritan Hospital for eight days and treated with antipsychotic medication. The doctor told my family I had postpartum psychosis, and I started receiving electroconvulsive therapy (ECT). It is not like it is portrayed in the movies. I was put under general anesthesia so there was no discomfort. It is supposed to affect the hormones and brain chemistry while putting the body into a temporary seizure. I still don't quite understand how a controlled seizure can be safe and effective for treating mental illness. I read somewhere that this regimen of so many treatments could possibly even help one to avoid taking medications. That's not why I was going however. I just wanted to silence my thoughts. I would hear voices and talk to people who weren't there.

I had ECT treatments at the same hospital on an outpatient basis. The doctor who did them would do it on Mondays, Wednesdays, and Fridays. I would get there at 6:00 A.M. and leave from the recovery room. I had a total of ten treatments, and the voices never completely left my mind. I was terrified before each dreadful treatment even though I was doing them voluntarily. The nurses were kind. They knew each person by first name as they were wheeled in and out. I think they assumed each patient having treatments was a little embarrassed. As my consciousness along with my dignity left the room, I felt completely helpless and at the hands of the anesthesiologist, the doctor, and the ECT nurse. Waking up in the recovery room, I was left with a pounding headache that would not leave for at least 24 hours. I lost a decent chunk of my life, too.

The treatment affects memory and has left me with a gate that just doesn't open. The first three months of Thomas's life are difficult to piece together. One of the stays in the hospital is a complete blank. I ask my husband and my mother a lot of questions. I am constantly asked if I can recall a certain time frame, and I am truly tired of telling people that I just don't remember. My memory has not made a grand entrance, and I don't think it will ever return. It is gone. All I have is pictures and other people's recollections of the last four months. My mind and body have shifted back into reality, and I am left with a severe depression. Some days I wonder how I can go through all of this and remain alive.

PART IV: THE PRESENT

I am still having obsessive thoughts. I'm a mess. I cannot work and am on Social Security Disability income. I feel helpless, hopeless, and lonely. I feel out of control. I have had changes in my medications and still do not have relief. I do not feel any different. I want to run away, but there really is nowhere for me to go where I would feel any different. My mother takes care of my son. I don't know what I would do without her. She helps out so much.

My nightmares are my obsessive thoughts. My obsessive thoughts are my nightmares. I can't watch movies; they put ideas into my mind.

I still am not interested in sex, although I love my husband very much. He is so supportive. But I feel sad all the time.

I hate the way I look. I gained 80 pounds during the pregnancy. I have gone on a diet now, and it was because I had finally had enough of myself in the mirror.

I feel like I have not bonded with Thomas like I should have. My mom has a tremendous bond with him that it so strong it makes me jealous. She says I shouldn't be, but I can't help it.

I now feel like I am going two steps forward and four steps back. I feel like soon I will see the light at the end of the tunnel. I think the new medication is starting to work. It is not supposed to have as many side effects so weight gain may not be an issue on the new medication. I am finally starting to lose weight as well. I have good days, partial good days, and bad days—but I may finally be getting better. I still attend the postpartum depression support group. Being in the same room with other women with the same illness continues to tell me I am not alone.

This is a disease. I have to keep telling myself that. I am not going to be better overnight just because I am starting to feel better a little bit every day. I am not to blame, either. This is not my fault. In the future, I will look back on these days and be truly grateful that I have support going through this. That is important for my recovery.

For those who love me, thank you for being there and understanding what this disease is all about. I will be back to feeling like myself again, I promise.

PART V: EPILOGUE

I received a letter from Eva about a year after she sent me her story. She reminded me of what she had been through and she wrote the following:

In January of 2005, I quit the ECTs. Amazingly I started getting better. I am no longer paranoid, depressed, or hearing voices. The obsessive thoughts have left as well. I feel like a new woman. I have my life back, and a new Eva has emerged. I just knew I would come back one day. And so did my husband. We are very happy right now.

Chapter 8

Obsessions and Delusions: Wanda's Story

First of all, to give you my background, I was raised in a Christian home. I had a great childhood with a loving, supportive family. I have always had many friends and have been a very positive person. I have never dealt with depression or any type of mental illness before I went through postpartum psychosis. And I have not since.

I married my high-school sweetheart (we were both voted "most popular" in high school). We always dreamed of the day we would raise a family of our own. I had my first son in 2000. When he was born he had a few problems. Immediately after his birth I felt strange and paranoid. I thought that something was wrong with me or the baby. I honestly thought I was dying. I had never felt that way before, and it soon went away after I started nursing him. I mentioned it to my doctors, and they didn't know what to make of it.

With my second baby boy, I had a wonderful birth with no complications. When he was three months old, I experienced full-on postpartum psychosis. It was a life-altering experience.

Thanksgiving night 2003, I found myself obsessing over a problem with my husband. I started to look into the things people were saying as if they were trying to give me a message. I couldn't sleep or eat for four days and I could feel that something was wrong. I felt paranoid about many things. I thought my husband had drugged me and had put cameras up in our house. I thought people were framing me to look like a bad mom so they could take away my kids. I also became very frightened that someone was planning to murder me. I was so obsessed with these irrational thoughts that I could hardly do anything I easily did on a regular day—get my boys dressed, fed, diapers changed, etc. I had to talk my way through it just to complete the task.

My family was concerned about the way I was acting, so my sister took me to the ER. Once there, I told them my mind wasn't working right and requested a drug test to see if my husband had drugged me. I filled out questionnaires and felt like every question was a test or was prying into my subconscious. They sent me home with an anti-depressant. By the time I got home, my mother had arrived. By then, my irrational and delusional thoughts had intensified. I started to think my mom and my husband were evil. I thought they were trying to keep me in this world which was literally Hell. Every time I looked at my three-month-old baby he would just grin from ear to ear at me—but I thought he was an angel. My husband and mother saw that I was getting worse so my mother tried to get me to take the pill they gave me from the hospital. My mind started churning with horrifying thoughts—I felt like my life was at stake. I ran out of the house, screaming at the top of my lungs for help, "They are trying to poison me! Call 911!"

They restrained me and took me back to the ER. On my way to the hospital I hallucinated that they were taking a baseball bat to me and beating me to death. That put me in a catatonic state for hours. I had the most horrifying, scary thoughts enter my mind. They decided to take me to a psychiatric hospital. So, I was loaded into an ambulance.

It was then that I started to think how evil everyone was and how anything that had substance or was of this world was evil. I thought the devil was jumping around from person to person. If someone was talking—the devil was in them. The people in the ambulance kept mentioning they were taking me to the hospital. But I believed with all of me—almost as though it was pure KNOWLEDGE—that they were literally taking me straight down to hell. I thought as soon as we arrived, I would be in hell forever. I felt like the only way I could save my soul—and the people who were possessed by the devil himself—would be to get up, take the steering wheel, and roll the ambulance until it killed all of us and we would be freed from this evil world. And I would be in heaven with my Heavenly Father and Savior, and they would be so proud of me for overcoming Satan. As I went to roll the ambulance and "save us," I discovered I was (LUCKILY!) securely buckled in and couldn't move.

Had I been anywhere else I am frightened to think what horrific outcome would have taken place. I am sure I could have been one of those "depressed moms" who just "got tired of her kids" and ended things tragically instead of seeking the help she needed, like Andrea Yates. That is why I am telling my story. More needs to be done, and more awareness is crucial.

I was fortunate to make it to the hospital and receive anti-psychotics and a wonderful psychiatrist to talk me back into reality. I was sent home after a week and a half. I still struggled with many more terrifying and horrible thoughts. I fought it for months but had a wonderful supportive family, husband, and mother to help. Especially my mother, who felt this might just be that "postpartum psychosis" she once heard something about.

I am back to feeling whole again. My oldest son is now three and my baby is twenty months. I am back to teaching school with my pre-schooler, attending play groups and church, making play-doh, and the other million things stay-at-home moms do. As I look back it is so hard to believe this actually happened—until I remember the scary reality I thought I was in.

I have been blessed in my life. And I was blessed to have my family together after something that could have been very tragic. I feel like it is my duty and my calling to share with others so more will be done for women and their families who suffer through postpartum psychosis.

Chapter 9

Suicidal Thoughts, an "Evil Dog," and a Call to Police: Nicole's Story

I am a 32-year-old mother of four children, ages twelve, eight, three, and ten months. I was hospitalized for postpartum psychosis.

I suffered from post-traumatic stress disorder for a long time, due to severe trauma in my childhood from years of incest. I had been psychotic before, when I was seventeen and had a miscarriage after being raped. At that time I was hospitalized for two months in an adolescent hospital. I had postpartum depression after the births of my first three children (all boys). But I did not know about postpartum psychosis.

In addition to the events of my past, I was dealing with a variety of life-stressors when my daughter was born. My father and my father-in-law, both, and a friend of mine died. (I learned of my father's death three days before my daughter was born.) My oldest son's father has bone cancer in his spine. My wedding anniversary is on September 11. And we were in the middle of moving.

I am an educated woman. I have my bachelor of science degree in journalism. I work for a major communications company. I want the public to be more aware about postpartum psychosis.

It was approximately six months after my daughter was born that I first exhibited symptoms of psychosis. It started with the worst migraine of my life. I have had severe migraines for 6 years but none like the one which occurred on April 24, 2002. It was as if I was being smashed in the back of my head with a hammer. I went to the hospital and started feeling very strange. My husband had brought our baby with us to the hospital and was in the waiting room. I kept hearing her cry, so I asked the nurse if my husband could come in the ER. She finally brought him in, with my daughter—who had not been crying at all. I asked my husband if she had been crying and he said no. There were no other babies in the waiting area.

There was a patient in the next room who had a severe cough and was a heavy smoker. (We were separated by a curtain.) The doctor came in to explain to her the situation ... then, it seemed to me, the same doctor came in on three separate occasions to tell her the same diagnosis and treatment.

I kept watching the clock, which was in front of me on the wall. Time seemed to stand still, and a few minutes seemed like an hour. I was given Demerol, and I had to be walked to my car—I felt drunk.

As the days went on, my symptoms grew worse. I thought my kids were all sick with some weird virus. My son looked jaundiced and very ill. I kept both of the older children home from school and took them to the doctors three times. The doctors said there was nothing wrong with the kids. I thought the doctors were wrong, and I kept looking in my medical book for an answer to their mysterious illness. My daughter had red rings around her eyes and she looked deathly pale.

My three-year-old son kept saying he was a monster and drawing pictures of bloody people. I kept telling him he was not a monster— only a little boy. I thought he was playing games with my head. He seemed to be laughing at me, manipulating me. I accused my older son of plotting against me—it seemed like he and my husband were in on some big secret and no one was telling me.

When I was having hallucinations, I thought my husband was playing tricks on me. Later, I was convinced in my own mind that he had turned the children against me. I felt that I was going crazy and I was helpless. It seemed like everyone was either staring at me or laughing at me. I couldn't watch TV because I thought they were talking directly to me. It seemed like time would just stand still. Five minutes seemed like an hour, and I would just keep watching the clock. There would be messages on my answering machine, and I never heard the phone ring.

One day I took a nap and when I woke up everyone in my house was gone. (My husband decided to take the kids out and let me rest, but I was convinced that they had all died.) I raced through the house looking for them. Every time I went to use the phone, there would be no dial tone. Finally, they came back and I accused my husband again of trying to make me feel crazy. He had no idea what I was going through and neither did I. He said it sounded like I was on some kind of bad acid trip.

I kept having flashbacks about my father molesting me. It didn't help that the Catholic Church scandal was constantly on the news. I believed that I predicted the Catholic Church scandal in 1988, when I had confronted my father about my half-brother molesting me from the time I was five to when I was nine years old. I had told him that priests were child molesters (in a letter) and he said, "That's like saying all the men in the navy are gay or all single mothers are prostitutes." After remembering about that letter, I was convinced that I was the "chosen one." God had chosen me to deliver a message to the world. (I am a Protestant, and I grew up going to church, but haven't been to church in eight years.)

I had paranoid delusions and thought the police were going to come to my house at any moment. It was a frightening situation, and I didn't have any idea what was going on. A few days later I was having trouble falling asleep. I was tossing and turning—I'd had complete insomnia during the entire pregnancy. I kept thinking about things like when I would die and how. I woke up my husband and told him I could not sleep because if I did, I wouldn't wake up. He was very annoyed with me and wanted to go back to sleep.

I went downstairs into the bathroom and looked at myself in the mirror. (My hair had been falling out, which is a common occurrence after delivery.) I was convinced I had cancer and that's why my hair was falling out. I looked like an old woman in the mirror. I noticed lines under my eyes I had never noticed. I started picking apart all the wrong things about my face and feeling disgusted with my looks. I wanted to get plastic surgery and fix everything. But then I thought if I was dead, I wouldn't have to get plastic surgery.

I went into the kitchen and got a pen and a piece of paper. I started to write a note to my husband—that I loved him very much, and I wanted him to take care of the kids for me. I talked about each child individually and pointed out several things I loved about them and how they made me feel. I knew I'd never see them again. I put the note in the bathroom drawer by the sink, so my husband would find it during the move. (We had just bought another house.)

I went back upstairs and woke him up again. I told him that there was something wrong with me, and I needed to go to the hospital. He didn't take me seriously and got mad because he had to wake up in a couple of hours to go to work. (He didn't want me to go to the ER because then he would have to take a sick day, and he was nervous that people at his job would be mad.)

I went back downstairs and got the suicide note and ripped it up. I was able to think rationally for a moment and decided not to kill myself, but I knew I needed to get help fast, or I would be dead by morning. Finally, I convinced my husband to call for an ambulance. He told the EMTs he didn't know what was wrong with me. He had no idea what I was going through.

As they took me into the ambulance, it was raining heavily. I saw a police officer with his cruiser lights flashing, behind the ambulance. No one else saw him there but me. When I got to the hospital, I thought the EMT said there were animals parading down the street from the zoo. Then he was laughing, and the nurse started laughing too. The doctor came in to examine me, and I thought he said the other doctor died. Then he said he was on a diet. He kept talking about the diet he was on. I started to get paranoid again and started causing a commotion in the ER. I thought he was trying to trick me by saying he was on a diet to see if I'd say I was on a diet too. I yelled at the nurses and other hospital workers and accused them of being part of the police cover-up. (Meaning my husband was going to have me committed to a mental institution by using his police power.) I thought he was against me and was making me think I was crazy. That he had this plan to get rid of me. I was convinced he had married me just to have me locked up.

Later, when I was home again, I began having suicidal thoughts on a daily basis. I also had thoughts about drowning my infant daughter. I had strange thoughts about God—thinking I was an angel and the Virgin Mary.

Then one day I thought that my dog said in a strange voice that she was an evil dog—that was the day when I called the police on myself and said, "I think there's something wrong with me ... my husband won't wake up." At that time, I had put my six-month-old daughter on the kitchen floor. I saw the dog go up to her and scratch her face with her paw (nails). My daughter started screaming. I picked her up and saw big gashes in her face. I ran upstairs to tell my husband, who was asleep. He woke up and said there were no marks on her face. I thought he was tricking me again. I told him I had called the police. I wanted to go to the hospital, but he wouldn't let me.

Then I kept running up and down the stairs—then he was asleep again. I wasn't sure if my husband had ever talked to me in the first place. Then I saw my three-year-old son on the steps with blood all over his hands. I thought he was a monster covered in blood. I asked him if his father was sleeping. He told me he was dead. When the police came, I let them in. I thought I had killed my whole family. I was crying and acting hysterical. My husband came downstairs to see what was going on. I thought it was his ghost. I asked the policeman if he saw my husband. He said "yes."

I was holding my daughter, and she looked dead. I saw tears in the policeman's eyes. I wasn't sure if he was even there, so he said I could touch him to see if he was real. I thought I was going to jail. I thought that they were just letting me hold my dead daughter so I wouldn't get upset. I couldn't believe that I had killed my whole family! I was very scared and thought about that woman Andrea Yates. I was afraid of what people would think of me.

The police said they were taking me to a crisis center. I was very paranoid and felt they were tricking me. They thought it would be better if my husband (who is a police officer and those officers were his coworkers) took me to the crisis place. Once I got there, I felt better, but I had a feeling I was being watched. I noticed video cameras in the room. I thought my husband was going to have me put in a psychiatric hospital and have me committed. I tried not to sound crazy and remained calm. I tried not to talk and just sat in a chair and closed my eyes. I felt a little better, knowing that my kids were not dead. But then, I kept imagining that maybe they weren't really there.

Finally, I spoke to a woman about what I had been feeling and seeing. I felt paranoid that maybe they would think this was Munchausen's, and I was trying to hurt my kids. I thought that they were going to investigate us and say we had been abusing the kids. About an hour later, they decided to take me via ambulance to a psychiatric hospital. I agreed to go and wanted to know what I was going through. I felt like I was losing my mind. I couldn't care about my husband or what he might think. (He had been dead-set against me going to a hospital earlier on during my postpartum psychosis.)

Anyway, the EMTs came in, and I saw one of them with a book that said *Your Worst Fears Come True* in his hand, and he showed it to me. I was put in the ambulance, and I thought I saw my husband following the ambulance. Then, I told myself that it wasn't him, and then he changed into someone else. At the hospital, I was greeted by a familiar-looking woman named Kathy. Then, I had the bizarre feeling that I was at the gates of heaven. I whispered to the woman that I had killed my family. She put me in a room and told me to completely undress. I was put in a gown and told to wait.

A woman came in and asked me some questions. She told me I wouldn't be judged here, but she only had five minutes to talk to me. I thought it was time for a confession, so I confessed to her everything bad I had ever done in my life. She just smiled and asked me to join her in a meeting with other people. I asked her if I could wear a cross around my neck, and she said yes. But I gave up my diamond earrings, diamond rings, and watch because I wouldn't need them where I was going. Then I heard them say the "DOC" was arriving, which I thought meant Deptartment of Corrections. I thought someone said it was my husband.

Then, I realized that he had killed me and the kids, not the other way around! That I was in heaven, and he was at the gates of heaven, but he was going to be given another chance. I was convinced that another patient at the hospital was my husband, but it was my job to find out who he was. If I could convince him to confess his sins to God, then we would all go to heaven together!

But then I was interrupted by a beautiful girl ... I was convinced I knew her. I asked her name and she said it was Christy. Then I was convinced she was one of my lost babies (from previous pregnancies— I have been pregnant 11 times!) I grabbed onto her and told her that I loved her. She said she loved me too, but she had to go back to earth. I cried and was taken away by some people in white coats.

I was put in a quiet room. I was convinced I was the Virgin Mary, and I had lived my life on earth as a human—a regular person. That's why I had to go through all the sexual abuse, rapes, and abusive relationships with men. I took on all that abuse, and I still believed in God. I started to cry tears of joy. I was so happy that God had seen everything good I had done in my life. I had raised my children well, put myself through college, and done well in my life, despite all the bad.

I spent three days in the quiet room. I knew I had to go through a test—I had to make all the patients at the hospital believe in me but not tell them who I really was. I believed I was the messiah—I thought I was getting all these messages from God. I thought my psychiatrist, who was an Indian woman, was God. She smiled at me and told me everything was going to be okay and that I would see my husband. Then my husband came into the room, and I asked him if he had watched TV at all (because I was convinced that everyone in the world could see me). He said he was Saint Michael, the angel. Then I realized that I had married an angel, and he had been testing me all along! He said I couldn't tell anyone but that we'd be together soon and that I had to get through this. I spent eleven days in the hospital trying to help the other patients.

I was put on Zoloft, Ativan, and Risperdal and Haldol (I had a severe allergic reaction to Haldol and had to be given Cogentin to counteract it). I could hardly stay awake. I thought they were trying to send me back to earth and trying to make me forget who I really was. My thoughts were very bizarre but everything I thought—I believed.

I thought that workers in the hospital were my dead relatives. Everyone in the hospital looked familiar to me—it was one big déjà vu. But the tests kept getting harder, and I had to convince a hospital worker, who was sort of mean, to confess her sins to God, and she would get to heaven. I thought that the hospital was the gateway to heaven and that all the patients didn't know that they had all killed themselves, and if they just confessed their sins to me, they would go to heaven.

After about a week, I started feeling better. I guess the medications were finally working. I know that what I went through sounds completely insane! But it all happened. I know it wasn't real, but even after I came home from the hospital, I thought I had a near-death experience.

My husband had a real hard time because he had to take nearly a month off of work to help me with the kids because I was in no condition to take care of them. He had taken care of them when I was in the hospital for eleven days. It must have been hard because I had been breastfeeding my daughter exclusively, and she had to be fed formula for the first time. My husband had to wean her, and all she did was cry. I had been the primary caretaker of the kids, and he sort of took it for granted. He didn't know much about how hard it was to take care of a baby, let alone three other kids!!

I think he has a true understanding now of what I went through, but he doesn't want to talk about it. I never paid much attention to the Andrea Yates case until I went through what she did. She had religious delusions also, and I think she had no idea what she really did at the time. I think she had been on antipsychotic drugs, but her psychiatrist had taken her off of them. I don't think she should be in jail. I think she needs psychiatric help. I know most people don't understand her and think she should have got the death penalty. Even with that mother Susan Smith—I think she may have had postpartum depression and that may be why she killed her kids. I know it's very rare to have postpartum psychosis, and I have never met anyone who went through it. Women don't want to even admit they had postpartum depression, for fear that people would think they were crazy or bad mothers. I know I had postpartum depression with the other kids too, but it wasn't as bad as this.

I know now that my husband was very scared of what I was going through and had never heard of postpartum psychosis, except for Andrea Yates. I think my husband was embarrassed of me acting this way and thought it would get back to his job and people wouldn't understand.

I did call Jane Honikman and Sonya Murdock of Postpartum Support International (PSI) while I was going through the psychosis. They offered a lot of encouragement, and it helped a lot. I think they saved me—they talked to my husband about postpartum depression and postpartum psychosis and said I needed to get to a hospital. That's why I became a member of PSI.

Chapter 10

Visions of Mother and Child "Cut Up": Lisa's Story

My name is Lisa, and I'm twenty-four years old. My daughter Megan has just turned one and is such a blessing to my life. But the journey we took to get here was long, dark, and at times horrific. Although this was a postpartum disorder, there were signals during my pregnancy. I had a wonderful pregnancy and felt such joy knowing that I would soon be a mom. I had an image of this perfect life ahead of me where everything would fall into place. There would be no lack of sleep or irritability, and each night I would have a clean home and wonderful dinner on the table for my husband. As my pregnancy was nearing its end, I started having frightening dreams. In one, I had just delivered my daughter, and the doctor dropped her on the floor. I had it over and over, sometimes the scene would change, and I had dropped her or a family member had dropped her. And even though I had worked in schools and had been a nanny for families with young children, I suddenly felt I wouldn't know what to do.

Then the day came, August, 2004, she was born. Suddenly I knew exactly what to do and was so in love with this little person. We went home, which was ninety miles away from both my and my husband's families, and started our new life. The first week was like any other new mom's. Steve, my husband, stayed home and helped us adjust. Megan only liked to sleep in my arms, so we slept in the living room so I could be in the recliner with her. As the weeks passed I found myself suddenly crying over nothing. Steve would go change Megan and come back to find me sobbing. I kept making excuses that it was my family being so far, or not knowing anyone in our new town, but it just kept happening. Still, I was so in love with Megan, I felt like she was my night and day, nothing else could compare to how I felt for her. After the first couple months my husband asked if I had PPD (postpartum depression), but I said no because I always wanted to be with Megan. And I thought you only had PPD if you didn't want to be near your baby.

I had also started seeing images. They were quick but horrible. I would see a man standing at the end of our hallway and then he was gone. I would also look up and see Megan thrown against the wall and falling down to the ground. It wasn't like I was doing it, but I saw it happening. I didn't want to say anything because I thought, I don't know, I just didn't know why anyone would want that to happen, and I didn't want anyone to think I wanted that to happen to my daughter. I loved her and was a good mom. Why would I want her to be hurt? About the same time these images started, I started having panic attacks. I would be driving and suddenly feel like I couldn't breathe and would start to cry. It was so frightening I didn't know what to do.

Unfortunately the frightening things didn't stop there. Megan was nursing every couple hours so I was awake every couple hours. She slept in a cradle next to our bed, and when I would put her back in, I was convinced that I had hit her head on the cradle. I was so afraid and felt so guilty because I thought I hurt her. Fears started emerging in other ways too; I was afraid that I would hit her head on the wall when I walked through the hallway. I was so afraid that I would walk further and further from the side each time. Again, I never told anyone—not even my husband or my mom, who is a labor and delivery nurse. I just thought it would all pass. The months went on, and I was still crying, having panic attacks, images, and fears. I was still doing everything a mom should. Megan was taken care of; we read books, sang songs, had tummy time, and even got out of the house for errands and trips. I was overly prepared, and trying to do everything perfectly. Megan always had on a cute outfit, and I always had my hair done and makeup on. Well, at least when we were out. At home I barely showered, always wore my pajamas, and never opened the door when a neighbor would come by. I did manage to keep things clean and dinners made, but they would have to be done in spurts, everything at once. Then I would be so exhausted I couldn't do anything more.

November and December came and were so busy. It seemed like we were rarely home; every weekend we packed everything up and visited our families. As much help as it was, it made life exhausting. Before Christmas we went on vacation with my family and I noticed another fear. I was afraid to go out on the balcony with Megan; I thought I might drop her off it. The whole time I avoided the balcony and couldn't understand why I thought I would drop her off. I knew I didn't want to, but I had a feeling that I was just going to do it. We returned home, and I felt that I should talk to my doctor about why I was still crying. I figured it would be something small and very easy to fix. The day after Christmas my husband left on a business trip, and I was getting ready to go home. At the same time my mom had talked to a doctor at her hospital about my crying, and she became worried that it might be more than I thought. After Steve left, my aunt asked if I was happy to go home, and although I don't remember it, I said I was "scared to death." That sent up a red flag, and my mom immediately made appointments for me. I didn't tell her what my visions were, but I told her I had some disturbing thoughts. We went to the breastfeeding (BF) clinic at her hospital, and I took a PPD screening tool, where they ask you a series of questions and you rate them on a scale of strongly agree to strongly disagree. Well, I "passed." The nurse told my mom not to leave me alone and to make an appointment with a psychiatrist. My doctor checked my thyroid, which came out fine, and I went to see a psychiatrist who didn't understand PPD, the visions I had, or the extreme fears that plagued me.

My visions had gotten worse; I was seeing images of myself and the baby cut up. It wasn't as if I was cutting the baby or myself, but it was happening to us. I would try to get the images out of my mind but I just couldn't. I was afraid to be near knives and razors. I still didn't want to tell anyone what I saw, but I did say I was afraid of sharp objects. I couldn't walk upstairs with the baby because I was afraid to drop her over the railing, so I would stay close to the wall and hold her as tight as I could. The next week I had a horrible panic attack in the car, and my mom had to come home from work. I saw the nurse from the BF clinic again who recommended to my mom that I be hospitalized. We felt I was okay but needed to be monitored, and my doctor said that was fine, and we'd know when it was time to go. For the first time I started to become distant from Megan; I wasn't interacting as much. My arms and legs felt so heavy; I thought I couldn't hold her, and although I was still nursing, I mostly pumped and fed her with a bottle.

Then it hit. . . . I felt like I was enveloped in darkness; I was nonresponsive to Megan and my family. I felt alone, like I was falling into a black hole. But this was only the beginning of the darkest days of my life. The next day I became incredibly afraid and paranoid. I started seeing things. Worse than before, I was seeing people walking upstairs and thought they were trying to get Megan. It was so real; I could see and feel that there were people trying to get into my house to kill my baby.

My mom noticed that something was wrong, and when I told her what I was thinking, she immediately took me to Las Encinas, a hospital that had a program for depression and psychosis. The last thing I said to my sister as I left was "don't let anyone in the house, they want the baby." PPD and PPP are very serious; however, there aren't many programs for recovering moms. Las Encinas was a good place for me to get on medication and get started on treatment. Although it wasn't a picnic, the doctor gave my family special privileges and allowed them to be there from the time I awoke to the time I went to bed. That was very important to me—as I was still very paranoid. I thought the patients wanted to kill me and that people were hiding in the bushes watching me. I was even afraid to use some of my toiletries as I thought they had been tampered with, and I didn't talk to anyone. My answer for everything was, "I don't know."

The doctor who was treating me seemed to have some sort of understanding of PPP; unfortunately, he was only on call for the doctor assigned to my case, who said I "should be back to normal in a week, not needing any kind of family support, taking care of Megan as usual." By the end of the week the psychosis was less, and the anxiety, although still prevalent, was better. Although I should have stayed longer, my desire and the view of the doctor pushed me to go home. I went home to my parents and started the next step of recovery. My daughter stayed with my in-laws as I still needed twenty-four-hour care, and my mom took family leave of absence. We used every resource her hospital had and found an amazing psychiatrist and therapist, both of whom understood PPP and the path we were on. I didn't speak much; sometimes it was as if I didn't know the words I was about to use. I was like a stroke victim. And I didn't want to be alone. I would follow my mom around or have her call my sister so I could hear her voice. I would go to appointments but couldn't talk; my mom or Steve would have to talk for me. I was just an empty shell.

After a month I was doing better, and Megan came home. I couldn't take care of her yet, but I didn't need as much care as before. Then about a month later my therapist recommended a doctor that worked with moms with PPD and other hormonal disorders. He ran some tests and found that I had no progesterone, and although my thyroid came back normal before, the T3 and T4 parts of my thyroid were also very low. After a few days of natural progesterone and thyroid care I noticed a huge difference. I was able to do more, my psychosis and paranoia were gone, and I was participating more in life.

Seven months later and we've still had ups and downs. Nothing as drastic as when I was hospitalized, but nothing like life before PPP. I have recovered quickly, say my doctors. For that I'm grateful to God, my family, and my doctors. I still can't handle too much stress, and get bouts of depression and anxiety, but I'm just thankful to be alive and to have Megan and Steve alive. Right now we're looking at the possibility of me having Bipolar II or soft Bipolar, as most women don't have PPP without an underlying precursor. And we have noticed that although I've had an amazing recovery, I still have a cycle of drops into depression. Some more severe than others but none that should just be lived with.

It was so difficult for me to find anyone that understood exactly what happened to me, and I don't want any other woman to feel as if no one understands. Please know that you are not alone, and that even though it feels as if you'll never get through this, you will. The things you experience are horrific and frightening, and you don't have to give people details, but you should tell someone there is something wrong. Without the help of doctors, medication, and family support, you won't be able to get through this horrible time. Don't be ashamed; you didn't cause this. It is in no way your fault, and it doesn't make you a bad mom, wife, or person. You are strong and brave for reaching out for help, and deserve to enjoy your baby and life. My deepest sympathy and prayers are with any woman who has to suffer through this. To the family members and doctors that read this, you are so important in these women's recoveries. I know it's hard, and there is so much you feel you don't understand, but just being there, encouraging and supporting them helps so much. Having someone to sit with so you don't feel alone is a huge key, and being told it's not your fault is very healing. Making sure that everyone involved is on the same page and has breaks is important. But most of all, just being educated on what's happening and knowing you will all get through this is the most important.

Footnote: Now, nine months after my hospitalization and thirteen since Megan was born, I finally feel normal. This past week I've been able to do two things I haven't been able to do until now: I can wake up with Megan if she has a problem at night, and I can wake up with her in the morning. This seems so small—but in recovery they're huge. Last night I was with her a lot as she was pushing through a molar, and this morning I woke up and thought, "Wow! This is what this past year was supposed to feel like." I'm not sad—as if I missed out on it all—although I did feel that way before. Now I'm happy. I feel like things have clicked, and I'm now able to fully enjoy life and motherhood. I was always told that I would eventually feel normal, but it is hard to imagine when you are in the middle of an emotional tornado. I now know what they meant about life suddenly clicking back in. And now I feel comfortable telling other women that they too will eventually feel like themselves again.

Chapter 11

A Maze of Medication and Recovery: Marti's Story

As I sit here and try to decide what to say and where to start with my postpartum story I am suddenly aware of why this is so difficult—I still (four years later) find myself very afraid of taking my mind back to that time, somehow thinking it might manifest itself again. However, here I go.

Looking back I realize how unprepared I really was for the birth of my daughter Beth. Sure, I had the perfect nursery; the clothes picked out; the birth announcements ready to mail; a cook, cleaner, and even afterbirth nurse to help; however, nobody ever told me about the emotions you would feel after giving birth, the intense hormonal changes your body would experience, how sleep deprivation could set in and take a toll on you like no other, and especially what changes transpire between you and your partner.

I was not married when I found out I was pregnant; however, I had a great job, a great partner, and an amazing family and set of friends, so I knew there was no way I could terminate this pregnancy. My partner and I spoke about marriage; however, we both agreed we did not want to do it just because I was pregnant—so we made the decision to undergo this adventure as best we could, supporting each other the best way we knew how.

As nine months quickly passed, I felt completely ready to give birth—I felt like my body was in the best shape it had ever been in, thanks to months of prenatal yoga and eating well. I was thrilled with the decision of selecting a doula to help us during the birth process. We met with her and laid out exactly what we wanted my birth plan to look like—"no medications" was at the top of my list. Not only was I scared to death of the epidural, but I was in a place at my life of no medications, organic foods, and homeopathic remedies for any aliments I had.

The birth of Beth could not have gone any better. I secretly hoped for a Monday morning birth (so I wouldn't be disturbing my doctor or family in the middle of the night) and out she came around two o'clock Monday afternoon, and through the support of my partner and doula, I gave birth without any medication.

I suspect the minute she was born I thought something was wrong—I didn't want to see her. I couldn't believe I just completed the most amazing physical feat I will probably ever endure, and I wanted my family, friends, and doctor to relish me with love, glory, and congratulations; instead all I felt was Beth got everything, and I was left with nothing.

The next week passed by in a daze of visitors, learning how to breastfeed, change a diaper (since this was the first baby's diaper I had ever changed), and trying to sleep.

The morning my partner had to go back to work after being off for a week was the point I knew something was drastically wrong. I was overcome with a fear unlike any I had ever experienced, and I could not stop sobbing. In the meantime I decided to start a journal of every time Beth ate, slept, and went the bathroom. I was suddenly obsessed with all her behaviors and schedule.

One afternoon my nurse said she thought I might be experiencing postpartum depression and recommended a therapist in the area to go and talk to. After my first meeting with the therapist, she immediately recommended I start a small dose of antianxiety medication—there were even ones compatible with breastfeeding. I thought about this but decided to try another route—I would see an herbalist and acupuncturist, and use vitamins, diet, and any other natural remedies I could find to stop these feelings of utter panic, anxiety, and obsession racing through me.

Another few weeks went by, and I was becoming increasingly worse inside, although I was very good at hiding it. Nobody knew I had written out plans for my funeral, down to each song I wanted played. I sold almost all of the stock I had from my previous employer, got all my other financial affairs in order to the best of my ability, and even began writing goodbye letters to each of my family members. I never once thought of harming my daughter, but surely the solution to this pain I was experiencing and the right thing to do was to end my life. I was not going to be a good mom, I was not going to be able to handle what raising children would bring, I had never loved something so unconditionally and intensely that it would be impossible to live without her, so I would make sure I left in case I ever had to experience the pain of life without her. All these irrational thoughts were constantly running through my mind.

Finally, after a visit to my doctor, I received a prescription for an antianxiety medication. Unfortunately, it did not work on me as it was meant to. My partner was leaving for a business trip for two days, and I knew I could not be alone. I took Beth to my dad's house where he and his new wife took care of her. I took my first dose of medication and within twenty-four hours felt like somebody had slipped me speed. I could not shut down the racing thoughts in my head, and I felt as if electrical currents were racing through my veins. At this point I had been without sleep for almost forty-eight hours and could barely keep any food down.

I remember leaving to pick up my partner at the airport, and I suddenly had to pull off the road and call my therapist. Once I reached her she gave me the name of another medication that would surely induce sleep and calm me down, as well as the number of a psychiatrist who I truly owe my life to. I don't really remember much after that—I remember my partner got into the car and immediately asked what was wrong. I couldn't tell him because I didn't know. As we drove along the freeway I remember rolling down the window and needing to feel the wind on my face—that was going to be the last moment I felt alive. I immediately tried opening the car door to jump out. I remember fighting with my partner to let me out and then grabbing the phone to call my twin sister. I needed to tell her goodbye.

I don't know how we got home; so many images and thoughts were racing through my mind, I couldn't focus on anything. My partner said he took our daughter to the neighbor's house, and while he was gone I called my dad and his wife asking to talk to my baby brother—I too needed to say goodbye to him. They tell me I said something about a gun, which is why the police were called. I remember hearing sirens approach our house, and I ran outside through the garage. As I was running around the corner knowing exactly where I was headed—the bridge up the street— two police officers grabbed me and put me back into the house.

I remember my dad and sister showing up, and my dad did not want them to take me to the hospital; he wanted to wait until we could see the new psychiatrist. It was decided that my dad would take Beth to stay with him and his wife—I never imagined it would be almost a month until I would be with her again.

I was given medication to try and help me sleep, but that is when I started having hallucinations. I was speaking and making no sense at all and felt like I was going to crawl out of my skin.

I woke up feeling like I hadn't slept a wink, although they say I slept at least seven hours. I was caught by my sister in the bathroom, cutting my hair and continuing to say things that made no sense at all. That's when the decision was made to take me to the hospital—for my own safety. I was admitted to the psychiatric ward on a seventy-two-hour watch. I could not believe this was where I was—a new mom struggling with her life, needing to be nurtured, reassured, and safe; this was not a place for postpartum sufferers.

I got out after twenty-four hours; I convinced the woman doctor who came to see me that I was having baby blues and just needed some sleep. In the meantime my partner had gotten through to the psychiatrist; however, we could not see him for one week. He did, however, prescribe for me more medications to get me through the week.

My partner needed to see and be with Beth, so we moved into a hotel near my dad's. While he spent as much time with Beth as possible, I existed in what felt like a comatose state due to the medication I was on. I suppose looking back that was the only way to keep me alive—existence in a state of nonemotion or feeling.

My appointment came with the psychiatrist, who immediately prescribed a new concoction of antianxiety, depression, and bipolar medications. I was also asked to attend a month-long voluntary program through the hospital to deal with anxiety, depression, and other mental health ailments.

We decided that until the medications began to work, it would be best for me to stay away from Beth. My partner took the next two months off of work and became an at-home dad while I moved in with my sister.

It seemed like it took years to feel better. I remember calling my psychiatrist and telling him if this stuff didn't work soon, I wouldn't be here much longer. He switched some things around, and within a few days I was starting to feel better. I remember listening to music, and it was a joy again—not an irritating, static sound. Food suddenly smelled good and tasted well. I suddenly wanted to see Beth and, more importantly, touch and hold her.

I am one of the lucky ones to have made it through what seemed like hell and back. I would not be here if it weren't for the amazing doctors I had, the postpartum support group where I live, and the love and support I had from my family and friends. I will continue to share my story and remain active as a member of the postpartum health alliance; my wish is that someday all women suffering this disease and their family members are able to get the help, resources, and support they need. I, too, hope all women suffering this disease will have the courage to speak up about it and ask for help—it is nothing to be ashamed of.

Chapter 12

Acting Well but Wanting to Die: Sarah's Story

Throughout my life I have always been considered a "happy" person, and there are many times that I have felt that I have had an unbelievably fortunate life. Things have always seemed to have gone my way, from graduating from college with honors, graduating from physical therapy school at the top of my class, to meeting the man of my dreams and marrying him. Everything went great until I became pregnant.

I believe that my depression began during my pregnancy. What I recall most about the day I became pregnant are my feelings of nervousness and disbelief, rather than excitement, although we had been planning and trying for several months. During pregnancy, in accordance with what I now recognize as obsessive-compulsive disorder tendencies, I diligently watched what I ate—but I also obsessed about my weight (with which I never had a problem), my body, and the baby's health. I had two scares early on, cramping that sent me to the ER, and spotting that was confirmed to be benign by my OB-GYN. My pregnancy was complicated by marked swelling in my legs, and urinary retention, which I was convinced at one point was a sign that I had multiple sclerosis. Towards the end of my pregnancy, my blood pressure began to rise, and the OB recommended that I begin more frequent visits to her to monitor for preeclampsia, with which I was later diagnosed. I remember feeling somewhat numb when I thought about the baby during pregnancy, but I believed that I would bond with her after she was born, even though I had a difficult time picturing myself as a mother.

Four weeks before my due date, my water broke. My husband (Cal) and I rushed to the hospital, and I remember thinking that I hadn't had time to mentally prepare myself for the baby to arrive. Marissa was born nine hours later after two and a half hours of pushing. Before I was given the opportunity to hold her, she was rushed to the nursery to be put under an oxygen hood, as she was having some difficulty breathing. I was confined to my bed, as I developed preeclampsia during the delivery, and I was put on an IV drip for twenty-four hours. I was unable to see or nurse my baby during this time, so my husband videotaped Marissa in the nursery and brought me the recorder so that I could see her. Marissa remained in the hospital for almost a week, and we stayed there with her, with me unsuccessfully attempting to breastfeed while at the hospital.

When we finally were allowed to take Marissa home, I continued to have difficulty getting her to latch on to breastfeed. I was extremely anxious and preoccupied by several things, including the fact that Marissa was losing weight, her sleeping patterns (she had her days and nights mixed up), and the fact that my husband did not have a job, as he had been laid off several weeks before Marissa's birth. This anxiety resulted in insomnia after about two weeks. Although I couldn't see it at the time, it was actually a blessing that my husband wasn't working, as he was able to care for Marissa while I tried to sleep. After about six weeks, I began to realize the severity of my anxiety so I called my OB, who prescribed me Prozac (the first of many antidepressants that I was to try) and referred me to a psychiatrist. Although Prozac was one of the drugs considered safe to use while breastfeeding, I did not feel right nursing while on medication, so I weaned Marissa. I felt very guilty, and began to feel like I was a bad mother because of this and because of my lack of feelings for Marissa. Cal appeared to bond with Marissa immediately, which added to my guilt and made me feel that Marissa loved my husband more than me. I quit taking the Prozac after one to two days, as I felt that it made me a "zombie" and less able to care for Marissa. After seeing the psychiatrist, I was started on different medications for postpartum depression, anxiety, and insomnia. I went through Celexa, Serzone, and Zoloft, to name just a few. I researched the side effects of every medication I was taking, and was convinced that anything that I was feeling was a side effect of the medications. I kept going back to the psychiatrist and insisting on changing the medications, so none of them actually had time to take effect. In the meantime, my anxiety was worsening, and I was constantly obsessed with the fact that Cal did not have a job. I was certain that once he became employed I would be fine.

Cal finally began working when Marissa was approximately two months old. For a few days I was less stressed, then my anxiety returned, this time focused on my belief that something was wrong with Marissa, and my perception that our relationship was damaged because of my postpartum depression, so that she was unable to bond with me. I was convinced that Marissa had a neurological disorder. The pediatrician tried to assure me that nothing was wrong with Marissa, and even ordered an EEG to further put me at ease. But even when the EEG turned out normal, I remained unconvinced. I continued to have difficulty sleeping and was also unable to concentrate or remember details of activities from as recently as the previous day. Tasks such as reading, balancing a checkbook, or watching TV were impossible for me. I simply could not concentrate enough to comprehend what I was seeing.

My anxiety became so bad that my psychiatrist suggested that I begin day treatment at the local hospital. I went to day treatment for about two weeks, and I met others in the group with the diagnosis of depression, but none with postpartum depression. I began comparing myself with the others and realized that what I was feeling was different—I was not feeling sad, just numb. I began to believe that I was not really suffering from postpartum depression. I thought I just had made a huge mistake in having Marissa, because I was not meant to be a mother. I became somewhat delusional, believing that I was somehow different from everyone else in the world and that I was incapable of being understood. I feared that this would lead to eventual commitment to a mental hospital for the rest of my life. I did not confide this to the staff—I did not want anyone to stop me from my plan to end my life. I began to pretend that I was feeling better, so that I could be discharged. I told the psychiatrist that I was beginning to feel better about myself and my baby. I believed that *nothing* could help me. I carefully researched on the Internet how to commit suicide. I knew that if I didn't succeed I would end up hospitalized indefinitely in the mental ward.

I was discharged from the day treatment program on a Friday. The following Tuesday I dropped Marissa off at daycare, went home, and took a large amount of Ativan and Ambien, washed them down with rum, and climbed into a bathtub of water, hoping to drown when I passed out from the medication. Six and a half hours later my husband found me still alive but barely responsive, in a miraculously empty bathtub, and called 911. I was rushed to the hospital and spent two days in ICU before I was transferred to the behavioral health wing of the hospital—into the "mental ward" that I was trying so desperately to avoid. There I again encountered others with depression, but none with postpartum depression.

I continued to feel that it was impossible for anyone to understand me. My delusions extended to beliefs that I had never had any original thoughts, that I had never loved anyone, and that I had always been this way but had always managed to fool everyone throughout my life—until now that everyone could see that I was not able to be a good mother. No one could convince me otherwise, despite many attempts by my friends. Friends would bring me books about postpartum depression to try to show me that what I was feeling was not unusual, but I could see no similarities to what I was feeling in these books. (The descriptions in the books were nearly identical to what I had been experiencing up to the point where I began experiencing psychosis. But because of my mental state I could not see that.)

My husband was incredibly supportive during this time. He brought Marissa to visit me nightly. At first I told him everything, but as the days went on and I thought that I would be confined there forever, I began again to pretend to be better. I told the staff that I was glad that my suicide attempt had not been successful and that I was feeling better about myself and missing my baby. Although none of this was true, I eventually convinced the doctor to discharge me. I immediately went home and continued to research ways to end it all. I had no idea what I was going to do. I just knew that I couldn't live like this, and I could not ever care for my baby.

Four days later I called in sick to day treatment, packed a bag, and headed towards the Blue Ridge Parkway with intentions of jumping off of a mountain. I found that I couldn't do it—not because I didn't want to die—but because I was afraid of surviving, and the consequences of that. My car broke down on the parkway, and I was forced to call my husband and explain what had happened. (My thinking was so unclear I was unable to think of anything to tell my husband but the truth.) He immediately took me back to the hospital, where I was admitted and then transferred the following day to a university hospital about two and a half hours away. It was there that I was first diagnosed with postpartum psychosis. At this point I began to believe that I was indestructible—that I was somehow superhuman and unable to die. However, when the doctors approached me with the idea of electroconvulsive therapy (ECT) treatments I agreed—not because I had hopes of getting better—but with the idea that maybe I could die during the anesthesia.

I had four treatments. After the first one I felt the same but pretended to be much better, hoping to be discharged. I'm not sure after which treatment I stopped pretending and actually began to feel better, but I soon realized that I was beginning to look forward to going home to my husband and daughter. I was discharged the day of my fourth treatment—almost two weeks after being admitted—with instructions to continue taking the antidepressant Effexor and the antipsychotic Zyprexa.

ECT miraculously snapped me out of my deep depression and false reality, and over time I began to grow in love with my precious daughter. Now at nine months post-delivery, I am back to work as a physical therapist, back to socializing with my friends, and enjoying life to the fullest. Also, thanks to the continuation of the meds, I am not the highly anxious person that has been typical of me throughout my life. I occasionally stop and grieve over the "lost time" with my baby, and I am envious of new mothers who feel the immediate bond with their baby. But I realize that what I went through has not been in vain. It is my deepest wish that I can somehow help another woman who is going through this type of personal hell. To help her realize that although this cruelest of diseases robs women of some of the most precious moments of their lives, it *is* only temporary and soon she will begin to enjoy motherhood and experience the ultimate joy of relating to her baby.

Chapter 13

Seeing a Dagger, Hearing Voices:
Tara's Story

Tara was living in England when, after a scary and disappointing labor where her birth plan was not followed, Tara's baby was born. This is her story:

In three pushes, with the suction, Zoe was born. It really upset me that I didn't get to see it. I was also upset that my birth plan was not carried out. It all happened so fast for me that I didn't have time to remember to ask them for a mirror. After the pushing, I felt relieved for a few minutes until I started to feel pain—the episiotomy. The doctor never told me that he was going to start stitching. Then I had to ask for more anesthetic for that. The doctor said, in a condescending tone, that I was "a big girl." He had said this earlier as well. I felt like he was saying that I was fat. And I had just lost lots of weight previous to the pregnancy, and the staff never had problems with my weight gains, etc. So I felt offended by that. Well, that was done. My husband took pictures of me, which were so hideous. I looked awful. Some photos were showing a partially bare breast. I just looked and felt horrible.

The midwife let me go to the bathroom as I had to pee, even though I had most shamefully peed all over everyone and everything whilst delivering my daughter. The midwife said she would be right back to clean me up after she did some paperwork and would be back in about twenty minutes. She arrived after an hour, almost an hour and a half. I was grossed out and feeling sick for all the blood on the floor on the way to the bath and all. She said not to worry. I felt a bit happy and proud that I had got through it, even though I was traumatized and feeling very bewildered and scared inside. I figured it would go away in a day or two. I got upstairs then and had to ask for something to eat. Got a packaged ham sandwich, no cheese. There was a lot of fat on the ham. It wasn't that good. And there was an orange. That was all, after not eating all day and burning all those calories in the process. If I wanted anything else I was shown where the kitchen was to make your own toast and get your own tea. Bob had to leave sooner rather than later, hospital policy.

Zoe was so upset, crying so much. I was in a ward with three other mothers. Their babies were all boys and quiet. The nurse took my baby from me right away, for a rest, and then brought her back, too soon because she was crying. The staff showed me how to breastfeed, but it wouldn't work when they left the room. One nurse gave her formula on the first night. I saw it on the cart. When I asked about it, she replied, "Well you don't have enough to feed her now, do you love?" I felt so inadequate and phoned my husband crying. He brought me a McDonald's breakfast the next morning, but otherwise all there was to eat at the hospital was corn flakes, packaged juice, no pulp, and toast and tea—all of which you went to get yourself. The staff would watch the babies in their nursery, and you could have a shower but someone would always trigger the alarm, and I would feel anxious and hurried to get my shower done quickly. The bath was a community bath, and we were told we had to clean it before using as anyone could use it. I only had two visitors—Bob's eldest brother and niece stopped by for five minutes with a card. I also got flowers from a neighbor, but no one else came to see me.

So, after three days of lousy meals and no rest we left to go home. I went in a taxi with the baby, and my husband went home in his work van. A neighbor asked me in for a minute, and then we were home. It was a bit cold in the house, and I went up to go to the bathroom. I came downstairs feeling shaky and told my husband that I didn't feel right. So, here I was home with this baby, who had colic, right away—every night starting around 5:00 P.M. She needed to be moving all the time, and wouldn't sleep for hours at a time. I kept calling the States, mainly to my aunt and some to my mother. Nothing worked. I tried breastfeeding. I wasn't sure she was getting enough, as my milk didn't come in for about five days.

My husband had off the first two weeks, and then the bad stuff really happened, although it started before he returned to work. I started getting scary images, hallucinations. Every time I looked up at the TV, I would see a dagger dripping with blood. I was also hearing a voice say to smother the baby. I would keep changing the voice to say "love the baby" or "soothe the baby." It was so tiring, fighting the messages all day and night. I thought about killing myself so I wouldn't hurt her. I kept planning these trips in my head, where I would go on the train to the Irish Sea and drown myself. I thought about going to the hospital and just returning her to the nurses and running. I was afraid to be near an open window with her, and even thought about pushing her into traffic while walking to the doctor for her checkup. I wasn't getting any sleep the first three weeks.

The crucial night came when I phoned the hospital late at night to say I couldn't do the breastfeeding anymore. I was practically hysterical. The nurse asked if I wanted to come back and be admitted to the maternity ward, and I said no. She also said not to bottle-feed because I would be feeding my baby rubbish. She called back later to see if I was okay and started again telling me not to give Zoe formula. My health visitor came by and said in her opinion, I should bottle-feed. That made me feel so much better. I was in no state of mind to decide things. Even when we brought her home, the midwife, Pam, extended her amount of visits. She was worried about us because the baby wasn't settled, and I was a mess. After a few weeks my fear was still there. Then guilt set in—I began thinking that my daughter would feel that I didn't love her or that maybe she would find out some day that I felt the way that I did, and she would hate me.

I made myself get out of the house and even went to a National Childbirth Trust meeting of other moms and babies. I didn't feel welcome there. Nobody ever called or asked to meet for lunch or even took my offers. I had phoned La Leche League about the breastfeeding. I got brochures, but no human being to be with me and help. No one to be my friend. Neighbors offered to watch her while I slept, but I felt self-conscious because she cried so much. I declined help.

I went back to Pam during the first couple of weeks after the birth for counseling. She could give me ten sessions, and then I was on a waiting list for more permanent counseling. After about two sessions, she was away on vacation for three weeks. I felt like I was hanging by my fingertips. Then, before the baby was seven months old, we were going to the States to see family at Thanksgiving and to have the baby baptized. I had to keep calling to see when I was going to receive counseling because the former was just temporary assessment, and I was on the NHS waiting list. [NHS is the National Health Service, free in the UK and Europe.] The issue was that Pam was a counselor for pre- and post-natal but only for a short-term counseling service. They fit me in with a woman for a few sessions, and then I had to wait about four months after that until I saw a really great counselor.

However, after I returned in early December from our Thanksgiving holiday, I sought out a daycare recommended by the health visitor. It was paid for by the borough, the local council. The kids were taken care of upstairs with education and caring, and the parents were taken care of downstairs, with cups of tea and information and conversation. A break, a time out. This and meeting a friend with a baby girl three months older than mine helped me on the road to recovery. Also, when my daughter was five months old, my fibromyalgia became bad. The doctor prescribed an antidepressant for it, and that also helped a lot with sleeping, rest, and better functioning of my joints, etc.

Regarding risk factors for postpartum depression, I had been married before and had been treated for depression, agoraphobia, and panic disorder. I was never on medication, but prior to meeting my current husband and having my daughter, I had made a good recovery after nine years and was leading a pretty active, happier life. Now it's difficult again because of this postpartum depression, to be strong and confident again. The other thing that helped me was going to the Internet and reading about postpartum depression, knowing there were others like me, and that I could recover. I liked Robin's Nest on About.com. There are great chat rooms and so much information. Really helpful. I had met several women who did my hair at a local beauty college in England who have had postpartum depression and still don't feel recovered fully, even years later. Each one encouraged me that I would feel better, but it could take about eighteen months. I feel for the most part that I should have had immediate help, maybe even hospitalization. I won't have any more children, primarily because of my postpartum experience.

PART III

Tragic Conclusions

I wanted this book to primarily be a book of hope and healing. However, tragedy is a very real risk of this illness, so I felt it was imperative that it be portrayed as well. The first of these tragedies is a story of suicide. I interviewed Carol Blocker, mother of Melanie Blocker Stokes, for this first story. Although, for obvious reasons, the experiences of those who commit suicide are difficult to fully portray, Carol generously offered portions of Melanie's diary to illustrate, as much as possible, what she was experiencing. Carol also provided a number of letters from women who wrote their stories for her and told her she had permission to use them. I've included excerpts of some of those with Melanie's story to further illustrate this illness.

The second story is an infanticide. It was written from prison. Many women are currently serving time for acts done while in the grip of this illness. Their stories could easily fill a book. Fortunately, there are women who have committed maternal infanticide while ill who have been tried by more sympathetic courts and have received treatment and not simply punitive incarceration. Some women have even succeeded in regaining custody of children that survived after they completed treatment. I had hoped to include one of their stories here. For obvious reasons, however, those women tend to be reluctant to share details. One of these women is considering sharing her story publicly after her child is grown. I hope she does; it is so important that we see these women as potential contributors to our community. We must become more interested in learning from these women for the purposes of prevention rather than simply punishing them.

Chapter 14

A Murderous Illness: Melanie's Story

This is Melanie's story, as told to me by her mother, Carol Blocker. The words in italics are direct quotes of Carol's comments from our interview.

When Melanie Stokes become pregnant, she seemed to have everything in place. She was a successful pharmaceutical sales manager happily married to Sam, a physician. She had a supportive family and her share of brains and beauty. She was a radiant pregnant woman, eager to meet the child inside of her and to begin her new life as a mother. On February 23, 2001, Melanie's daughter, Sommer Skyy, was born. Sommer was a beautiful, healthy baby. But Melanie's mother, Carol, realized right away that something wasn't quite right with her daughter. Melanie, who had dreamed all her life of holding her baby girl in her arms, did not seem to know how to respond. Although Carol was worried, she convinced herself that the labor had exhausted Melanie, and that when Melanie recovered she would return to her normal self. But Melanie didn't bounce back.

I knew something was wrong as soon as Sommer was born. There was so much going on during the birthing, I did not notice anything. But as soon as Sommer was born, Melanie went flat-line. She was not responsive. They gave her the baby. Her husband asked, aren't you happy?—or something like that. She gave a small smile but did not say much. I told the doctor that something was wrong. The doctor said they would keep her another day.

When asked, Melanie denied that something was wrong. Sommer was born on a Friday. That Saturday, Melanie could not get herself together. When Carol brought balloons, Melanie did not even thank her—which was unusual. Melanie was irritable. She did not focus on Sommer at all. She just sat listlessly on the edge of her bed. Carol called her sister and said, "Something is wrong."

Melanie and I were extremely close; I picked up on it immediately. A mother knows her child.

Melanie was not her cheerful, happy, normal self, although even during labor she had been happy and cheerful.

Before this, Melanie had always been bright and sunshiny.

When Melanie went home and Carol asked what was wrong, Melanie said she had a lot going on physically. The next day Melanie said she made a big mistake. She said she was going to put Sommer in day-care the next day.

If I had heard of postpartum psychosis, I would have known it from her symptoms.

Melanie said that Sommer did not like her. Sommer was probably four weeks old at this time. Melanie insisted that Sommer responded to Carol and Sam but not to her. At this point, Melanie's depression had grown so severe that she had stopped eating and drinking and could no longer swallow. When Carol saw that Melanie would not drink or eat anything, Carol insisted that she go to a doctor. Melanie said that the doctor did not like her—did not even want "to see her face."

Not long after that a knife was found in Melanie's bathtub. When Melanie was asked about it, she said she was not sure what she was going to do with it yet. Melanie told her mother, "Don't bring me any more presents, and I don't want any more company."

I was bewildered and I hurt for her. I told her, "I don't know what has happened to you, but we will get through this." I told my sisters that I thought Melanie had had a nervous breakdown. I thought that the labor pains must have been too much for her.

By then, Melanie, the Melanie I knew, was gone.

Melanie began to have paranoid thoughts about others—she thought that her neighbors across the street had all closed their blinds because they thought she was a bad mother. She became gaunt, hollow-eyed, a shell of her former self. Then, she began searching for a way to end her life.

Her brother called me at work to say, "There is something wrong with Melanie." She had just called him and asked him to buy a gun in the projects. I left work and went to her and chastised her for it. I took her to the doctor's office and said, "Melanie is thinking about killing herself." He asked her, "What are you going to do?" She replied that she had thought about carbon monoxide.

Melanie was hospitalized three times in seven weeks.

The first time she was hospitalized it was for hunger and because of her comment about carbon monoxide. She was put on medication to improve her appetite. The medicine worked to improve her appetite, but she still thought of suicide.

She was cheeking her other medication. She was in the hospital for about a week. At one point she said the toilets in the hospital were so big you could drown yourself in one if you wanted. I called the hospital and told them about that and they said they would move her bed to the hall if necessary. They said they would watch her.

When she came home, she was eating but still talked about suicide. About the second night she was home, Sam woke up and realized

Melanie was gone. When he went out to look for her, he saw her coming back from the lake.

It was around this time that she stopped talking to me.

Melanie went to a neighbor and asked him for a loaded gun. The neighbor told Carol to take Melanie's talk of suicide seriously.

I was shocked. At that point one of my sisters came over to watch Melanie every day.

One day, Vera, Carol's sister, was sitting with Melanie when Melanie requested to go shopping to get birthday presents. Vera asked why; the birthday Melanie was talking about was not until November, and it was still April. Melanie said that she would not be around by then.

Melanie said that Sam and Sommer would be better off without her because she was a terrible person and terrible mother. Melanie then told Vera to take her to the train station to get a schedule for a trip Sam was going to take.

That trip for Sam—that was completely fabricated.

Vera took Melanie to the train station. Melanie got out and went in while Vera stayed in the car. Then it dawned on Vera what Melanie might do so she leaped out of the car and ran into the station—so quickly that she left her purse behind. She saw Melanie by the tracks. Vera ran to Melanie as fast as she could. Vera asked Melanie what she was doing, and Melanie said "nothing."

The next day, Melanie wanted to stay around Carol's house and Carol's sister Grace's house. While there, Melanie began to fixate on the windows and began taking the screens out. On the way home, Melanie started having chest pains.

Now I know that was probably an anxiety attack. At that point Melanie had been home about a week. We realized we could not watch her adequately so we decided to take her back to the hospital. I tricked Melanie into going by saying that the doctor said that they had given her the wrong medication, and it was causing her high blood pressure. When we got to the hospital there were no rooms available, so she was taken by ambulance to another hospital.

On Monday, Melanie was seen by her doctor. She was given medication that takes about two weeks to work.

The nurse told me that Melanie was not taking her medication, but that there was nothing to do about it; the hospital has an honor system about taking meds. At this point all Melanie communicated to me was hopelessness, saying things like, "Nothing is going to work," and "I have no choice"— death talk.

Melanie was released on Friday.

I tried to talk to her doctors, but the psychiatrist said she could not talk to me and told me not to call her anymore.

I knew she was no longer Melanie. But no one would talk to me about what was happening. No one would say what was wrong or whether they had seen this before.

Melanie was admitted to the hospital a third time.

She began writing crazy things in her notebook. She wrote journal entries asking if she had done something to offend God.

ENTRIES COPIED FROM MELANIE'S DIARY, PROVIDED BY CAROL

Undated.

How can I explain to anybody how something has literally come inside my body—took away my tears, joy, sleep, ability to eat—drive function at work take care of my family.

Sam, Mom and Dad are so sad. I miss everyone! Sooo much. I'm just a useless piece of rotting flesh. no good to anyone. no good to myself.

Undated.

Sam can't understand how a person who has everything could not want to do all the stuff of life. No one can truly understand.

I WANT MY LIFE BACK

I don't want, didn't choose to be this way.

This life now is No Life at all!

Hocus Pocus is for real

Why did this have to happen?

Undated

I have been sentenced and doomed to Live a Life

Without

Smiles

happiness

Love

Joy

Food

drink

work

my husband

my family

my baby

Without food my body eats itself.

This is the Supernatural

one day I wake up pacing then increasingly tired.

then disturbed[?] enough to go outside

then I feel the <u>thump</u> in my head.

My whole life becomes altered

Hell is the worst possible consequences of one of your choices.

Saturday April 2001
I have really tried to be a good recovery patient
No one else thinks so
I am sorry to cause so much pain.

Undated.
Please forgive me
> **Sam**
> **Sommer**
> **family**
> **friends**

When they admitted Melanie, the doctors told me they could not answer my questions due to the Hippocratic Oath. That was around Mother's Day—we had brought Sommer Skyy in to visit Melanie. But Melanie would not hold Sommer or anything. She had had two shock treatments by then but had refused the third.

Melanie refused to interact with anyone or attend the group meetings. She said she did not want any visitors, presents, anything. Melanie stayed in the hospital for a week and then came home. In addition to the electroconvulsive therapy, Melanie was given four combinations of antipsychotic, antianxiety, and antidepressant medications.

Carol was taking care of the baby at this time.

I told Melanie's father, "Don't let her come home—if you do—kiss her goodbye. If you cross the street, hold her hand, she wants to die." But no one took me seriously. Melanie had two personalities at this point—goody two-shoes for Sam—she tried to put on a good face (and with the doctor too)—but with me she was honest. I knew she was sick.

Melanie stayed home a week while Sommer stayed with Carol. She was listless, not herself.

She told me not to come over one day—a Friday—she said she wanted to spend some time by herself with her husband. But he went to a meeting and left her. Later, Sam said Melanie was having breakfast and smiling. Melanie called me and told me that Sam was taking a shower. I said I was on my way. But Melanie said Sam was getting tired of me. She said that to keep me from coming.

That day, Sam left for a meeting, and Carol did not come over. It was the first time Melanie had been left alone. Melanie took a cab and went downtown to a Day's Inn.

I don't know how she got a room. She didn't have any identification on her. She spent the weekend there—although we didn't know it until that Monday when she got up and did her deed.

When Sam returned home, Melanie was not there. He called Carol to see if Melanie had gone to visit Carol. They then informed the police that Melanie was missing and eventually gained press coverage over the weekend.

We called the police, searched for her, put out flyers. I picked up newspapers and called them and told a reporter about it, and they put it on the front page of the newspaper. Then it got on to the radio and television. I told them Melanie had had a baby and postpartum [psychosis] and was missing. The woman reporter said the newspaper would run the story because if not for her dad and the parish priest, the same thing might have happened to her mother.

I told my sister that Melanie was looking for the right time and place to kill herself. The black churches had prayer services—she was our star. We were popular here on the South Side of Chicago.

On Monday, I didn't know what to do with myself—so I went up to school. When I was walking up there a teacher ran up to me and said, "Oh Carol, your daughter just jumped out of a window." It had been on the radio. One of the teachers had heard it on his way to school, and he had told the other teachers. I turned around and went back home—I didn't know what else to do—I felt helpless.

All of my friends came over and started planning the funeral—the police and news media came—all the channels and even the Mexican channel. I talked to everybody.

The police went to Sam's house and showed him her clothes and took him and Melanie's father to identify her.

I couldn't go. I've never seen her dead. I couldn't see her in her casket—I could not do any of that. I could not put her in the ground—instead I paid the expensive price to put her in a crypt.

Over a thousand people came to Melanie's funeral.

Carol began going to every hospital in the area to ask, "What would you do if she came to you now?" She gave them brochures (from Depression After Delivery) and started giving talks at hospitals. But she doesn't feel as if it has done much good.

Carol wrote Oprah and got on her show. She wrote to everyone she could think of including the cardinal, the surgeon general and the governor of her state. The responses she received often looked like form letters. Then Carol got a letter from Congressman Bobby Rush (IL) saying he wanted to introduce a bill for research. Carol continued to write letters—to the National Institute for Mental Health, to the Department of Health and Human Services, to (then) President Clinton and the First Lady.

I rarely heard anything back. Then I went to visit the girls in Dwight (an Illinois penitentiary) who had killed their kids—you would have thought that I was their guardian angel—they just hugged and kissed me.

Melanie is gone, but Carol continues her quest. Congressman Bobby Rush reintroduced the Melanie Blocker Stokes Postpartum Depression Research and Care Act (H.R. 1940). Each year women and children lose their lives to this illness. If you wish to help, you may contact your congressional representatives and urge them to support this bill.

The Melanie Stokes Foundation Web site (http://www.melaniesbattle.org) states, "Although Melanie's family rallied around her with all their strength, in the end, Melanie jumped to her death from the twelfth floor of a Chicago hotel."

Melanie's death left her family with many unanswered questions. Carol is angry at the doctors who did not seem to recognize the peril Melanie was in. She does not understand why she was not given the information she needed to help fight this illness. The Web site is her effort to get the word out about postpartum psychosis. She hopes that by sharing Melanie's struggle, she will raise awareness about this volatile, often misunderstood, illness.

The best way to contact Carol Blocker is by telephone: (312) 225-1310 or go to her Web site and leave a message on the board.

Carol has received letters from a number of women who have given Carol permission to use them as she sees fit. Carol sent that correspondence to me for use in this book. The following are some excerpts from those letters.

From a woman incarcerated for infanticide of a neonate conceived by rape: "Suddenly in my mind, I was a child and I had a doll that was never real to begin with. My whole world was upside down. I was in a state of confusion ... I knew I should not have a 'doll' because I was supposed to be grown up."

Another woman described her symptoms: "It was like watching a stranger ... a robot in a mommy suit." "I would see ... objects float by, just out of my peripheral vision, but when I turned to look at these things, they were gone." "I would have visions of disturbing violence, like [when] I stood at the bathroom mirror and 'watched' myself plunge a pair of scissors deep into my eye." "I found myself feeling like I was miles away, and not caring enough to 'come back.'" She concludes her letter, stating, "The diagnosis of PPD is still up for debate, but the actual depression was (and is) very real."

From another woman: "I thought of Melanie often during that time and thought she was lucky. Her suffering was over ... The intrusive thoughts continued ... I decided that going in front of a train would be the quickest and least painful way to do it ... That's when I knew I was seriously ill ... I was told I could not get an appointment for a month. A month?? When you finally decide to get help, you want it right then!"

This woman called a hotline and found help at a community hospital. A nurse there told her she would get better, saying, "It won't happen today and it won't happen tomorrow, but it will happen." She concludes her letter with, "I used to think that Melanie was lucky because her suffering was over. I now know that I am lucky because my suffering is over too. But I still have my life ... I feel like Melanie helped save my life. I know that there are many other women out there who need her too."

Chapter 15

Ninety Miles with a Dead Baby: Katherine's Story

When I first read Katherine's story, I thought she sounded eerily detached. But then again, her description of her experience conveys a rather surreal state of mind. The question that continues to haunt me about Katherine's story is: How could a woman in this condition be permitted to leave the psychiatric hospital, especially with a baby?

I was referred to Katherine by Postpartum Support International. She graciously responded to my request for her story. Katherine has been incarcerated since 1995 for the death of her infant daughter, Mylyssa. This was her reply.

I am reconstructing my story the best I can. My current mental health is stable—I still have *mild* mood swings due to menopause now.

Before my incarceration my hobbies were crafts (hot-glue), collecting sea shells and pine cones for decorations, gardening, hiking, camping, Bible Studies, cooking/baking, sewing projects, exercising, classical music and Christian music concerts, and shopping. I plan to resume these hobbies when I am released and off parole. Currently I garden a little and write articles, poems, and essays. I have had fifteen articles, poems, and essays published since my incarceration.

I am now 51 years old. (September 3, 1951, is my birth date.)

Here is my story:

I. MY LIFE PRIOR TO POSTPARTUM DEPRESSION/ POSTPARTUM PSYCHOSIS

I have a melancholic disposition. Throughout my teenage years and earlier adult life I was manic-depressive. I also suffered from PMS with severe mood swings and very heavy periods. I am very sensitive and internalize everything. I used to base most of "life" decisions—career, living locations, mates—on how I "felt," rather than on logic or reason.

During my younger adult life I had a few mental breakdowns with attempted suicide.

However, I was highly functional—I maintained the "veneer" of "performance" at church, on the job, with my friends and family. Socially, I'm friendly, but most of my life I've preferred solitude to a social gathering. Not because I dislike people, but because I feared being rejected by people.

II. MY EXPERIENCE OF POSTPARTUM DEPRESSION/ POSTPARTUM PSYCHOSIS

I was unaware of postpartum psychosis—I only knew of the baby blues, and little of that yet.

I made a bad choice—in 1989 I married a man who lived a very secretive and secluded life. Prior to marrying JR, I worked as a secretary/ clerk/receptionist. When we married, I stopped working to become a stay-at-home mother to JR's five-and-a-half-year-old son. JR did not want any more children and being that I was told in my twenties and thirties that I couldn't have any children, I didn't worry about it.

Until February of 1995.

Then at age forty-three and a half, I came up positive for pregnancy. JR was okay about it—but we already had six years of a stormy marriage with verbal and mental abuse. JR would throw things and destroy the house to terrorize me. He very seldom had steady employment. When I would go to church for counseling, all I would be told was to submit myself more to God and to be more submissive to JR.

Because of JR's lack of responsibility, I had to take second-rate medical care at a high-risk pregnancy clinic under Medi-Cal (state aid). I did not see an actual doctor until my seventh month of pregnancy. During my pregnancy I experienced high anxiety, especially from my fifth month on. I started withdrawing myself from church. By the time I was in my seventh month of pregnancy, I had totally isolated myself, afraid to go out around other people.

By that time, I even "suspected" the doctors and nurses were talking behind my back and calling me "the crazy lady." During several checkups I visualized my blood pressure cuffs "exploding." From my seventh month to childbirth I only went out to doctor's appointments and nowhere else.

My mother stayed with me from August 1995 to October 1995. Mylyssa Grace made her debut after an emergency C-section on September 26, 1995. Prior to her birth, I felt I may be dying. I had panic attacks. I felt like I was in a dark hole. I even had paralysis in my left foot that still exists seven years later.

A week or two before Mylyssa's birth, I had a terrible and strange episode. My mother could not wake me up—when the emergency team checked me for transport, my blood pressure had dropped to 60/ 30. Also, by now I distrusted everyone around me.

What happened after Mylyssa's birth was even worse. I ran away from the hospital, forgetting momentarily that I had just given birth to a baby and was attached to an IV pole. It took three officers to bring me back to the hospital. I was wearing only a hospital gown.

Why did I do this? Because I feared for my life. I felt that everyone was in a conspiracy to kill me, including all my friends, my mother, JR, my family, and all the nurses and doctors as well. First I was told by hallucinatory voices that the hospital staff would drain all my blood out into a gallon milk jug. Then the staff was going to cut all my bowels out by opening up my C-section.

Then later, while I was in the bathroom (after being disemboweled), the voices told me "they" would be poisoning me with carbon dioxide through the vents. Then my body was to be transported to the roof where the staff would throw me off the roof. The voices continued, telling me that after that, my body would be taken to the main oxygen control room where my body would be filled with oxygen to the point of exploding. These voices finished the "death scenario" with the "fact" that my body parts would then be vacuumed up so no one could ever find me. So, because I feared for my life, I "escaped" the hospital.

When I was returned, my psychosis worsened. I not only heard voices, I started visually hallucinating. I saw people "melt" in front of me. (I've never taken illegal drugs, etc., in my life.) I was seeing rooms tilt at weird angles and seeing people who were not physically present.

Because Medi-Cal only covered my six-week checkup for postpartum care, I only spent two days at a psychiatric care facility and was released. When I read my case file in prison, it indicates that my condition was inconclusive. And I could not find one shred of evidence referring to who signed me out of that facility. And I could find no mention of a plan for follow-up care.

At home, when well-meaning people came to visit me, I barely recognized them. I felt paranoid, even to the point that when friends brought food over during the first week, I thought that it was poisoned.

My mother helped quite a bit—I could barely take care of myself. The voices not only were telling me of a death conspiracy against me, but these voices at times suggested suicide as a way out.

In the meantime, my husband was nonsupportive. I vaguely recall an incident that my mother reminded me of. We lived in a semi-rural area near mountains. There was a fire in the mountains. As my mother tried to get me, Michael (my stepson—then eleven years old), and Mylyssa out of the house, JR acted abusively and wouldn't let us leave—stating that he didn't care if we all burned to death. Before my mother left to go home, she and JR got into a huge fight—she even had to have my friend take her to the airport.

Eleven days later I was still hearing voices. I still did not trust any-one. I felt alone. I felt that I wasn't a good mother.

November 11, 1995—Mylyssa wouldn't stop crying. I tried to rock her, burp her, change her diaper ... then I suddenly psychologically snapped. A voice told me that if I covered my baby's face to stop her crying that I'd be a good mother. I did—I killed the very precious child that was dear to me. (I also dearly loved my stepson as well—but Mylyssa was my own flesh-and-blood child.)

Because Mylyssa didn't turn blue right away, I at first thought she was sleeping. A few minutes later when I realized she wasn't moving, I tried to resuscitate her with mouth-to-mouth breathing—but to no avail.

JR called and said he would be home in five minutes. With his abuse, I feared for my life.

I put my child's tiny body back into her crib and covered her up.

JR came home, as did Michael from wherever he was playing. I made dinner and went to bed—thinking maybe this was just a bad dream and that maybe in the morning I'd wake up and find out it really didn't happen.

When I woke up early, about 5:00 or 6:00 A.M., I showered. Then I remembered we were going to church, so I thought I would check on the baby and get her ready. When I looked in her crib, and she was all blue, terror filled me. I took my dead baby, got into my husband's truck, and drove aimlessly down the freeway. I drove to a friend's house ninety miles away, but she wasn't home (she was at church)—so I left to go back. Much of this time in the truck remains very vague in my memory—I was in a zombie-like state as if I was detached from what occurred. I vaguely remember voices suggesting that I should die and try to get out of this life so I could atone for all the evil around me. On the way home I saw a gasoline tanker truck ahead of me. The voices told me to go ahead—end my life and everything would be fine. As I accelerated, the transmission of my truck went out, and I slowed down. God had a different plan for me.

I exited the freeway seven hours later, called my husband, and told him where to meet me. He showed up with a friend and they called 911. That is where I was arrested with my dead baby.

I was so scared. I'd never been in trouble before in my whole life.

III. MY ARREST AND INCARCERATION

My arrest and incarceration at Robert Presley Detention Center in Riverside, California, was very abusive. My first few days there I was put in a strip cell with no clothes, no sanitary pads (after having a baby), no bed, no blankets—just a makeshift rubber gown that kept falling off of me, exposing my naked body to male guards. I was given only one cup of water and two meals a day. I was told to eat off the tray on the floor like the "dog that I was" for killing my baby.

The sheriff's department ran my story in the Riverside *Press-Enterprise* newspaper. They lied. They said I deliberately killed my baby and that I even *said* I did it deliberately. In reviewing my case file in prison, I could not find any transcript that showed where I had made such a statement.

Interestingly enough, the only psyche report missing when I went to take my plea bargain eleven months later was the psyche doctor for the D.A. (district attorney) and sheriff's department.

Two male guards purposely told all the inmates, as I walked past them going to court, that I was a "baby-killing bitch." In prison I still am very much alone because of my case. I try to reach out to women like me—but they are very fearful to come forward.

IV. WHO I AM NOW

Basically, I'm the same person in a lot of areas. I still have my faith in the Lord Jesus Christ (I am a Christian)—as my personal Lord and Savior—as I did before this happened. However, this time in my life— the postpartum psychosis, Mylyssa's death, and the incarceration— have strengthened my faith in the Lord. I realize how much I've been forgiven, and how much the Lord loves me and knows I was mentally ill when this happened and that I truly loved my beautiful, red-haired, blue-eyed baby girl.

Who I am now is a woman—not only forgiven by God—but blessed with the love and forgiveness of friends and family who still support me. And I *finally* have forgiven myself.

I am also free of my abuser. JR turned out to be a closet drunk during our thirteen years of marriage. He also had women on the side, before and after my incarceration. He is now in Texas and plans to file for a divorce. I pray it will be soon. He has thrown out everything of mine—my clothes, photos, personal papers—everything I owned. I have nothing material left.

However, I have everything. I have my sanity restored. I have peace with God, myself and those who truly love me. I am more grateful—I love to celebrate life and live each day to the fullest. I give glory to God for restoring me to Him as my first love.

When I am paroled I will move to a Christian safe house for battered women coming out of prison. I am a woman who went to "hell" and back because—mainly—from a hormonal imbalance and secondarily because of a trauma from spousal abuse.

I give you permission to print all of this or whatever needs to be printed to help illustrate postpartum depression/postpartum psychosis as it relates to the postpartum experience that is "out of the norm," and also as it relates to the legal, medical; and judicial aspects in our society as well.

In a subsequent letter, Katherine said that she is divorcing JR on grounds of adultery, abuse, violence (including during pregnancy and postpartum), and abandonment.

I had written to her and asked what the people around her said or did about her behavior postpartum. She replied, "Not much—my friends and family at the time were very ignorant—as was I—about postpartum psychosis—its symptoms, its effects, and its treatment. I was pretty much "expected" to "return to normal" like "most women."

Chapter 16

Conclusion: What We Know, Don't Know, and Need to Do to Prevent Tragedy

When my publisher first suggested this chapter, I thought, "sure, that will be *easy*!" I anticipated this would amount to ten or fifteen bullet points per item and that would be that. But the more I thought about it, the less straightforward it seemed. There is conventional wisdom, and there is what we actually know. For example, conventional wisdom says one to three out of a thousand women who give birth will have PPP (postpartum psychosis). I was recently told that this number is based on scientific studies. But who is included in those studies? Are they all new mothers caring for their infants? How is "give birth" defined? Does it include miscarriages, stillbirths, or abortions? How do the researchers define postpartum psychosis? I've known several women who were diagnosed with "postpartum depression with psychotic features" whose symptoms look awfully similar to those with a diagnosis of "postpartum psychosis." How would those women be classified in the studies? How accurate are these studies? The more I thought about it, the more I felt there was very little we "know we know," a fair amount of "think we know" (conventional wisdom), and a fair amount of "know we don't know," or don't even realize we don't know.

Then I began to wonder, "Who is 'we'?" Is it postpartum advocates, the medical profession, outcomes from research? After mulling it over, I finally came to the conclusion that I am most qualified to say what the "royal we"—that is, "I"—know. So that is where I will start.

WHAT WE KNOW

- Without change, more children and mothers (and others) will die because of this illness.

- The rate of this disorder has been stated to be *"one or two"* or *"one to three"* *out of every 1,000 postpartum women will have PPP.*

- Although this is a very dangerous disorder (*3–4 percent risk of infanticide or homicide, 4–5 percent risk of suicide),* most women recover without harming anyone.

- Stigma about mental illness continues to make it difficult to speak openly about this. PPP is usually temporary. There are thousands of women in the United States who have suffered this illness and are now well.

- Lack of recognition in the DSM seems to have led to a lack of recognition of this disorder in medical practice and other areas as well.

- If a woman does not have a previous *diagnosis* of a disorder, she is not likely to be *assessed* for risk of PPP but may have *identifiable* risk factors and not know it. Even those with a previous diagnosis of a disorder, including bipolar disorder or PPP, are not always adequately informed of their risk nor offered preventative options.

- Women with PPP are often in the position of recovering from a stressful and strenuous event, often involving physical trauma or surgery, while caring for a newborn, and perhaps other children as well. That puts these women in a higher risk situation than a general onset of psychosis.

- Although this is not a new illness, it is easier for people to dismiss it if they can characterize it that way.

- This illness is not caused by laziness, wealth, poverty, abuse, or bad moral character.

- A woman who has had one (or more) child(ren) without becoming ill is not necessarily "safe" from this illness.

- Most experts agree this illness tends to occur in the first three months postpartum, often in the first two weeks.

- It is not always obvious that a woman is psychotic, and she may successfully hide it, *but* that does not mean she can control it. In addition, the intensity of the illness may change, giving the illness a waxing and waning quality that can be very misleading.

- There are very few absolutes to characterize a woman's symptoms. For example, she may know that what she perceives, at least some of the time, is not real, or she may not. She may have the ability to read, drive, reason, or plan, or she may not. She may be able to concoct elaborate lies, or she may not. She may speak of harming herself or her child, or she may not.

- There are doctors and experts who have techniques and treatments for evaluating risk and for preventing and treating this illness. This is not true for every doctor or expert.

- It has been recommended that PPP be treated as a bipolar illness until and unless that is ruled out. This means that prescribing an antidepressant, such as a selective serotonin re-uptake inhibitor (SSRI), may be counter-indicated as something that could cause more harm than good.

- Many women do not receive adequate care.

- Women with previous postpartum suicide attempts have been identified as higher risks for infanticide.

- Many women who have committed infanticide or suicide sought help first.

- Often those around these women—friends, neighbors, family—knew *something* was wrong.

- Even with support new parenthood can be difficult. Reality is not like the effortless, blissful myth of new motherhood. Without support it is almost certainly difficult. That difficulty is exponentially magnified by a mood disorder.

- Suicide and infanticide have been identified as natural outcomes of this illness when left untreated. Experts believe these are largely preventable with proper care.

WHAT WE DON'T KNOW

Of course there are things that we don't know. The following are things that we (I) *know* we (I) don't know.

- How much of an effect, if any, does past trauma have?

- What percentage of women could be accurately identified as at risk for the illness and prevented from having it?

- What form of initial treatment is the best? Do we currently wait unnecessarily long to use ECT?

- Does this illness occur at the same rate across cultures, races, and geographic locations?

- Are there various biological or genetic predictors for this illness? (Recent research indicates there probably are.)

- Do other physical factors play a role? Is so, how?

- Is PPP related to schizophrenia identifiably different from PPP related to a bipolar disorder? If there is a difference, does it have a significant effect on risk of infanticide or suicide?

- Are there identifiable variants of PPP that would indicate distinct causes, different rates of recurrence, a need for different methods of treatment, and differences in the fullness and speediness of recovery.

- Are there different risk profiles based on underlying disorders. For example, I have heard speculation that perhaps all or the majority of PPP-related infanticides are committed by women with underlying schizophrenic disorders. Of course, like other postpartum disorders, this might have a postpartum onset or be otherwise undiagnosed prior to becoming pregnant or giving birth. If this were the case it would call for much more aggressive screening to identify risk.

- Are there other/more/better methods of prevention? With adequate care could we prevent all *cases* of PPP and make this disorder essentially extinct?

- What is the connection between bipolar illness and PPP?

- Why does it happen to some women for some births, but not all births?

- Why do some women become suicidal, infanticidal, or homicidal and others do not?

- What percentage of women who experience command hallucinations attempt or commit suicide or homicide?

- What percentage of women who attempt or commit suicide or homicide experienced command hallucinations?

- Are the current statistics for rates of PPP, PPP-infanticide, and PPP-suicide correct?

- Can we accurately identify those with no risk of PPP?

- How many doctors know what steps to take to try to prevent PPP? Treat PPP? And how does the layperson find these doctors?

- What type of training, at a minimum, should family doctors, OB-GYNs, midwives, doulas, nurses, police, paramedics, and other professionals receive regarding this illness? What would be "ideal"?

- Are there different *types* of PPP?

WHAT WE NEED TO DO TO PREVENT TRAGEDY

Even this heading gave me pause. After all, if a tragedy is that which brings great harm or suffering, every experience of this illness is a tragedy. When we have tools for risk assessment, prevention, diagnosis, and treatment that are not used, many are *preventable* tragedies. When we have persons in authority who mistreat these women, it is preventable tragedy. The suicides, infanticides, and homicides that result from this illness are tragedies of almost unimaginable proportions. So, how do we prevent these tragedies?

- Official recognition of this illness, especially by medical, legal, and insurance professionals, as well as historians, academics, and media professionals.

- We must recognize this as a biological illness, not one *caused* by external factors such as bad relationships, dominating husbands, money issues, lack of education, or too little to do. These may influence a woman's mood, but they do not cause the psychosis. When we focus on those things we lose sight of the real problem.

- Education of the public: Family and friends are the first line of defense against this illness. They are in a position to notice the signs *if* they are aware of them and to seek help for the woman who likely cannot seek help for herself. Juries who are aware of this disorder are less likely to be misled by myths, biases, and stereotypes.

- Education of care providers: From OB-GYNs and midwives to pediatricians and family practitioners, we need to raise awareness of this illness and enable them to identify "red flags" that indicate a need to determine whether or not the woman is ill.

- Education of emergency workers: This includes police, social workers, ambulance, and emergency room workers. They need to understand how to handle a woman with a psychotic illness in a manner that will not put anyone at risk and will not needlessly exacerbate the woman's condition.

- Education of legal professionals: Prosecutors, judges, defense attorneys, and even guards need to better understand the illness from the woman's perspective so that their first exposure to this illness will not be in the context of a recent homicide.

- Screening and information: A woman has a right to know the *identifiable* risks she might face due to a pregnancy. When a woman and her medical providers are aware of potential risks, there is a greater opportunity for prevention. This is true of PPP as well. We should have prenatal and postnatal screening available.

- Prevention of the illness: Doctors need to know the methods and treatments of preventing this illness and offer them to their clients.

- We need more research on causes, prevention, and treatments. There are many promising possibilities, but we need further research.

- Effective and adequate treatment offered to all women who screen positive for a postpartum mood disorder.

- A society that values motherhood and parenting to the extent that it is willing to invest in it beyond lip-service. This includes safety nets for single mothers and their children.

- We must address the health of the mother in a context other than the health of the baby. "If mama ain't happy, ain't nobody happy." We cannot stop at "the child appears healthy and cared for" and assume that means all is well.

- Coordinated health care: We need communication between health professionals and an awareness and concern for the whole person, including family circumstance.

- We need mother-baby units where a mother can continue to bond with her child and know her child is cared for while she receives treatment. Too many families are tempted to act as though treatment for this illness is optional due to the logistics of childcare and the stigma of mental illness.

- We need databases of care providers who are trained to deal with this illness, and lawyers who are educated and willing. We need to be able to tell these women where they can get help: with insurance issues, with care for their child while they seek help, with custody issues, transportation, management of their symptoms, and treatment.

- We need a new specialization—experts specifically trained in women's reproductive mental health—both to identify reliable sources of care for these women and reliable sources of information on this illness within the legal arena.

- We must recognize that these women are those *least* likely to be able to prevent deaths associated with this illness. It is up to the medical profession, the legal profession, state and federal legislatures, and us, the public, to take responsibility for prevention.
- Legislation: We need laws similar to the British Infanticide Act that limit punishment and provide treatment when it is shown the woman has a disturbance of mind. We need passage of the MOTHERS Act and similar legislation to provide funding for research, education, and prevention.

THE GOOD NEWS

If there were promise of a vaccination against postpartum psychosis, would it be worth funding? There are treatments that show similar promise regarding prevention—it only takes our collective will to address and prevent this illness. Aren't our community's children and mothers worth it?

Remember:

These women are not alone (hundreds if not thousands suffer every year).

These women are not to blame (they did not choose or cause their illness).

There is help (there are effective methods of prevention and treatment).

They will be better (this is a temporary illness).

Notes

INTRODUCTION

1. (Rowling 1999, 82).

CHAPTER 1

1. (*Diagnostic and Statistical Manual of Mental Disorders IV-TR* 2000) (*Diagnostic and Statistical Manual of Mental Disorders IV* 1994).
2. (*Diagnostic and Statistical Manual of Mental Disorders IV* 1994).
3. (Sichel and Driscoll 1999, 242).
4. (Sichel and Driscoll 1999, 241).
5. (Sichel and Driscoll 1999, 244).

CHAPTER 3

1. (Pauliekhoff 1992).
2. (Dunnewold 1997, 1).
3. (Hamilton, *Patterns of Postpartum Illness* 1992, 6).
4. (Hamilton, *Patterns of Postpartum Illness* 1992, 7).
5. (Marland 2004, 32).
6. (Dunnewold 1997, v).
7. (See Hamilton, *The Issue of Unique Qualities* 1992).
8. (Hamilton, *The Issue of Unique Qualities* 1992, 16).
9. (Hickman and LeVine 1992, 284).
10. (Hickman and LeVine 1992, 284).
11. (Marland 2004, 209).
12. (Marland 2004, 4).
13. (Marland 2004, 4).
14. (Sichel and Driscoll 1999, 251).
15. (Marland 2004, 209).
16. (Hamilton and Harberger 1992, xiiv).

17. (The Marcé Society n.d.).
18. (Postpartum Support International n.d.).
19. (Davis and Stumpf 2008).
20. (Davis and Stumpf 2008).
21. (Postpartum Support International n.d.).
22. (Honikman 2007).
23. (March of Dimes 2007).
24. (Helzner 2008).
25. (Tibbetts 2008).
26. (Shannonhouse 2003).
27. (Shannonhouse 2003, 3).
28. ("The Yellow Wallpaper" 2008).
29. (Porter 2002, 239).
30. (Chesler, *Women and Madness* 1972, 48–49).
31. (Chesler, *Women and Madness* 2005, 105).
32. (Jones 1980, 55).
33. (Jones 1980, 55).
34. (Jones 1980, 55).
35. (Jones 1980, 57).
36. (Jewett 2004).
37. (O'Malley n.d.).
38. (Marland 2004).
39. (Marland 2004, 3).
40. (Marland 2004, 4).
41. (Marland 2004, 4).
42. (Marland 2004, 14).
43. (Marland 2004, 63).
44. (Marland 2004, 227).
45. (Marland 2004, 13).
46. (Marland 2004, 75).
47. (Marland 2004, 79).
48. (Marland 2004, 123).
49. (Marland 2004, 93–94).
50. (Marland 2004, 124).
51. (Marland 2004, 76).
52. (Marland 2004, 71).
53. (Sichel and Driscoll 1999, 240).
54. (Sichel and Driscoll 1999, 251).
55. (Birch 1994).
56. (Hrdy 1999, 294).
57. (Marland 2004, 14).
58. (Dunnewold 1997, 16).
59. (Pauliekhoff 1992, 247).
60. (Marland 2004, 202).
61. (Rynor 2008).
62. (Picard 2001).
63. (Mansnerus 1988).
64. (Martinez 2000).
65. (Elkins 2007).

66. (Mansnerus 1988).
67. ("Baby blues" defense successful in past cases 2001).
68. (Casey n.d.).
69. (Satel 2001).
70. (Marland 2004, 174).
71. (Spencer 2002, 36).
72. (Satel 2001).

CHAPTER 4

1. (Parnham 2008).
2. (Sichel and Driscoll 1999, 245–246).
3. (Johnson 1990, 326).
4. (Spinelli 2003).
5. (Parnham 2008).
6. (Perfect Storm 2008).
7. (Perfect Storm 2008).
8. (Spinelli 2004, 1552).
9. (Sichel and Driscoll 1999, 250).
10. (Kamisar, LaFave, and Israel 1990, 830).
11. (Kamisar, LaFave, and Israel 1990, 831).
12. (Parker 2006, 2A).
13. (Macfarlane 2003, 155–156).
14. (Macfarlane 2003, 155–156).
15. (Macfarlane 2003, 136) (See also Wisner, et al. 2003, 41).
16. (Macfarlane 2003, 136).
17. (See Wisner, et al. 2003, 44).
18. (Gado 2008).
19. (Spinelli 2008).
20. (Spinelli 2004, 1549).
21. (Katkin 1992, 275).
22. (Katkin 1992, 280).
23. (Kumar and Marks 1992, 262).
24. (Frith 2005).
25. (Frith 2005).
26. (Spinelli 2004, 1552).
27. (Spinelli 2004, 1553).
28. (Spinelli 2008).
29. (Johnson 1990, 301–302).
30. (Spinelli 2004, 1552).
31. (See Johnson 1990, 284–286).
32. (Marland 2004, 174).
33. (Parker 2006).
34. (Parker 2006).
35. (Johnson 1990, 287).
36. (Johnson 1990, 290).
37. (See Johnson 1990, 293).
38. (Spinelli 2004, 1555).
39. (Spinelli 2008).

40. (Martini 2006, 107–108).
41. (Spinelli 2004, 1553).
42. (Wolf 2003, 149).
43. (Wolf 2003, 149).
44. (Parnham 2008).
45. (Parnham 2008).
46. (Spinelli 2008).
47. (See Hickman and LeVine 1992, 289).
48. (Hickman and LeVine 1992, 286).
49. (See Hickman and LeVine 1992, 287).
50. (See Hickman and LeVine 1992, 286–288).
51. (Meyer and Oberman 2001, 86).
52. (Murdock 1987–2008).
53. (Murdock 1987–2008).
54. (Murdock 1987–2008).
55. (Night n.d.).
56. (Murdock 1987–2008).
57. (Murdock 1987–2008).
58. (Murdock 1987–2008).
59. (Murdock 1987–2008).
60. (Spinelli 2004, 1550).

Bibliography

"'Baby blues' defense successful in past cases." *Los Angeles Times*. June 24, 2001. http://www2.ljworld.com/news/2001/jun/24/baby_blues_defense/.

Beck, Cheryl Tatano, and Jeanne Watson Driscoll. *Postpartum Mood and Anxiety Disorders: A Clinician's Guide*. Boston: Jones and Bartlett Publishers, 2006.

Bennett, Shoshana S., and Pec Indman. *Beyond the Blues: A Guide to Understanding and Treating Prenatal and Postpartum Depression*. 2nd ed. San Jose, CA: Moodswings Press, 2006.

Bennett, Shoshana S. *Postpartum Depression for Dummies*. Hoboken, NJ: Wiley Publishing, Inc., 2007.

Birch, Helen, ed. *Moving Targets: Women, Murder, and Representation*. Berkeley, CA: University of California Press, 1994.

Casey, Laura. "Mother kills baby in suicide attempt." *Oakland Tribune*. http://www.findarticles.com.

Chesler, Phyllis. *Women and Madness*. Rev. and updated. New York: Palgrave MacMillan, 2005.

———. *Women and Madness*. New York: Avon Books, 1972.

Collins, Gail. *America's Women: 400 Years of Dolls, Drudges, Helpmates, and Heroines*. New York: HarperCollins Publishers, Inc., 2003.

Collis, Louise. *Memoirs of a Medieval Woman: The Life and Times of Margery Kempe*. New York: Harper and Row, Publishers, Inc., 1964.

Davis, Wendy, and Devani Stumpf. "PSI timeline 2008 update." Personal correspondence with author. July 2008.

Diagnostic and Statistical Manual of Mental Disorders: DSM IV-TR. Vols. 4th ed., text revision. Washington, DC: American Psychiatric Association, 2000.

Diagnostic and Statisticial Manual of Mental Disorders: DSM IV. 4th ed. Washington, DC: American Psychiatric Association, 1994.

Dix, Carol. *The New Mother Syndrome: Coping with Postpartum Stress and Depression*. New York: Pocket Books, 1985.

Dunnewold, Ann L. *Evaluation and Treatment of Postpartum Emotional Disorders*. Sarasota, Florida: Professional Resource Press, 1997.

Elkins, Lucy. "Baby blues made me cut my wrists." The Daily Mail, MailOnline. Associated Newspapers, Ltd. May 2, 2007. www.dailymail.co.uk/pages/live/articles/health/healthmain.html.

Frith, Maxine. "Scrap outdated infanticide law, say judges." *The Independent.* May 4, 2005. http://www.independent.co.uk/news/uk/crime/scrap-outdated-infanticide-law-say-judges-495016.html (accessed August 11, 2008).

Gado, Mark. "The insanity defense." *Crime Library.* Turner Broadcasting System, Inc. 2008. http://www.crimelibrary.com/criminal_ming/psychology/insanity/1.html (accessed February 29, 2008).

George Parnham, JD, criminal defense attorney, represented Andrea Yates. Interview by Teresa Twomey, JD. (August 5, 2008).

Halvorson, Shirley Cervene. *Beth: A Story of Postpartum Psychosis.* Bloomington, IN: First Books Library, 2004.

Hamilton, James Alexander. "Patterns of Postpartum Illness." In *Postpartum Psychiatric Illness: A Picture Puzzle,* edited by James Alexander Hamilton and Patricia Neel Harberger, 5–14. Philadelphia: University of Pennsylvania Press, 1992.

Hamilton, James Alexander. "The Issue of Unique Qualities." In *Postpartum Psychiatric Illness: A Picture Puzzle,* edited by James Alexander Hamilton and Patricia Neel Harberger, 15–32. Philadelphia: University of Pennsylvania Press, 1992.

Hamilton, James Alexander, and Patricia Neel Harberger, eds. *Postpartum Psychiatric Illness: A Picture Puzzle.* Philadelphia: University of Pennsylvania Press, 1992.

Helzner, Judith F. "Three pillars of maternal health: Low-tech, low-cost ways to save women's lives." *Ms. Magazine,* Summer 2008: 24, 25.

Hickman, Susan A., and Donald L. LeVine. "Postpartum Disorders and the Law." In *Postpartum Psychiatric Illness: A Picture Puzzle,* edited by James Alexander Hamilton and Patricia Neel Harberger, 282–293. Philadelphia: University of Pennsylvania Press, 1992.

Honikman, Jane. *I'm Listening. Spectrum of Postpartum Emotional Reactions.* www.janehonikman.com/imlistening.html 2007. (Last accessed November 15, 2008).

Hrdy, Sarah Blaffer. *Mother Nature: Maternal Instincts and How They Shape the Human Species.* New York: Ballantine Books, 1999.

Jewett, Thomas. "Patrick Henry: America's Radical Dissenter." The Early American Review, Summer/Fall 2004, Vol. V. No. 2. DEV Communications; Archiving Early America. http.//www.earlyamerica.com.

Johnson, Phillip E., ed. *Criminal Law: Cases, Materials and Text.* St. Paul, MN: West Publishing Co, 1990.

Jones, Ann. *Women Who Kill.* New York: Holt, Rinehart and Winston, 1980.

Kamisar, Yale, Wayne R. LaFave, and Jerold H. Israel, *Modern Criminal Procedure: Cases, Comments and Questions,* 7th ed. St. Paul, MN: West Publishing Co., 1990.

Katkin, Daniel Maier. "Postpartum Psychosis, Infanticide, and Criminal Justice." In *Postpartum Psychiatric Illness: A Picture Puzzle,* edited by James Alexander Hamilton and Patricia Neel Harberger, 275–281. Philadelphia: University of Pennsylvania Press, 1992.

Kumar, R., and Maureen Marks. "Infanticide and the Law in England and Wales." In *Postpartum Psyciatric Illness: A Picture Puzzle*, edited by James Alexander Hamilton and Patricia Neel Harberger, 257–274. Philadelphia: University of Pennsylvania Press, 1992.

Macfarlane, Judith, JD. "Criminal Defense in Cases of Infanticide and Neonaticide." In *Infanticide: Psychosocial and Legal Perspectives on Mothers Who Kill*, edited by Margaret G. Spinelli, MD, 133–166. Washington, DC: American Psychiatric Publishing, Inc., 2003.

Mansnerus, Laura. "The Darker Side of the 'Baby Blues.'" *New York Times*. October 12, 1988. http://www.query.nytimes.com.

The Marcé Society. *Mental health support for babies and their mothers*. St. Albans, UK. http://marcesociety.com (accessed November 15, 2008).

March of Dimes. "Professionals and Researchers: Quick Reference and Fact Sheets: Birth Defects and Genetics: Down Syndrome." March of Dimes Foundation, March 2007. http://www.marchofdimes.com/professionals/14332_1214.asp (accessed August 11, 2008)

Marland, Hilary. *Dangerous Motherhood: Insanity and Childbirth in Victorian Britain*. New York: Palgrave MacMillan, 2004.

Martinez, Renee, Ingrid Johnston-Robledo, Heather M. Ulsh, and Joan Chrisler. "Singing 'the baby blues': A content analysis of popular press articles about postpartum affective disturbances." *Women & Health*, 2000.

Martini, Adrienne. *Hillbilly Gothic: a memoir of madness and motherhood*. New York: Free Press, 2006.

Meyer, Cheryl L., and Michelle Oberman. *Mothers Who Kill Their Children*. New York: New York University Press, 2001.

Murdock, Sonia. *Postpartum depression legislation in the United States: A brief history*. Postpartum Support International. 1987–2008. http://postpartum.net/resources/healthcare-pros/legislation-history/ (accessed July 2008).

Night, Susan S. *A Missed Opportunity to Bring Change for Women Suffering From Postpartum Depression*. http://www.law.uh.edu/healthlaw/perspectives/2007/post-partumdepressionlegislation.pdf.

O'Malley, Suzanne. In print. *What the Critics Are Saying*. Suzanne O'Malley, The Official Website. http://www.suzanneomalley.com/publications.php (accessed July 31, 2008).

Parker, Laura. "The power of an expert witness." *USA Today*, June 21, 2006.

Pauliekhoff, Bernhard. "Toward the Diagnosis of Postpartum Psychotic Depression." In *Postpartum Psychiatric Illness: A Picture Puzzle*, edited by James Alexander Hamilton and Patricia Neel Harberger, 239–249. Philadelphia: University of Pennsylvania Press, 1992.

"Perfect storm." *Wikipedia*. June 30, 2008. http://en.wikipedia.org/wiki/Perfect_storm (accessed August 6, 2008).

Picard, Anna. "Could you too be a killer mummy?" *New Statesman*. July 9, 2001. http://www.newstatesman.com (accessed October 14, 2007).

Porter, Roy. *Madness: A Brief History*. Oxford: Oxford Univesity Press, 2002.

Postpartum Support International Web site. http://www.postpartum.net.

Postpartum Support International. "Rep. Rush's postpartum depression bill receives overwhelming support as it passes the house. *PSI News*, Fourth Quarter 2007: 13.

Poulin, Sandra. *The Mother-to-Mother Postpartum Depression Support Book.* New York: The Berkley Publishing Group, 2006.

Riklan, David, and Dr. Joseph Cilea. *101 Great Ways to Improve Your Health.* Marlboro, NJ: Self Improvement Online, Inc., 2007.

Rowling, J. K. *Harry Potter and the Sorcerer's Stone.* First scholastic trade paperback. US: Scholastic, 1999.

Rynor, Becky. "Infanticide is sadly not rare." *canada.com.* Canwest Publishing, Inc. June 21, 2008. http://www.canada.com (accessed June 25, 2008).

Satel, Sally. "Mommy undearest." *Slate.* July 4, 2001. http://www.slate.com (accessed October 14, 2007).

Shannonhouse, Rebecca, ed. *Out of Her Mind: Women Writing on Madness.* New York: The Modern Library, 2003.

Sichel, Deborah, and Jeanne Watson Driscoll. *Women's Moods: What Every Woman Must Know About Hormones, the Brain, and Emotional Health.* New York: William Morrow and Company, Inc., 1999.

Spencer, Suzy. *Breaking Point.* New York: St. Martin's Paperbacks, 2002.

Spinelli, Margaret, a leading writer, teacher, clinician, researcher and consultant on psychiatric disorders during pregnancy and postpartum. Interview by Teresa Twomey, JD. (July 2008).

Spinelli, Margaret. "Maternal infanticide associated with mental illness: Prevention and the promise of saved lives." *American Journal of Psychiatry* 9 (September 2004): 161: 1548–57. http://ajp.pyschiatryonline.org (accessed various times during Summer/Fall 2008).

Taylor, Verta. *Rock-A-By Baby: Feminism, Self-Help, and Postpartum Depression.* New York: Routledge, 1996.

Tibbetts, Graham. *Mothers' acute post-natal depression could be genetic.* November 3, 2008. Telegraph Media Group, Ltd. www.Telegraph.co.uk (accessed on November 5, 2008).

Wisner, Katherine L., Barbara L. Gracious, Catherine M. Piontek, Kathleen Peindl, and James M. Perel. "Postpartum Disorders." In *Infanticide: Psychosocial and Legal Perspectives on Mothers Who Kill,* edited by Margaret G. Spinelli, MD, 35–60. Washington, DC: American Psychiatric Publishing, Inc., 2003.

Wolf, Naomi. *Misconceptions: Truth, Lies, and the Unexpected on the Journey to Motherhood.* New York: Anchor Books, 2003.

"The Yellow Wallpaper." *Wikipedia.* Last updated November 5, 2008. http://en.wikipedia.org/wiki/Yellow_Wallpaper (accessed August 5, 2008 and November 5, 2008).

Appendix A: Resources for Further Reading

The first part of this appendix contains books, divided into categories. I've noted my "top 5" choices for the person who is seeking more information on psychosis and wants to get right to the point. These are the books that I return to again and again.

The second part of this appendix contains organizations and Web sites for further reading. Appendix B has resources for help.

ON POSTPARTUM PSYCHOSIS

Halvorson, Shirley Cervene. *Beth: A Story of Postpartum Psychosis.* (A mother's story of her daughter's tragic postpartum suicide.)

Marland, Hilary. *Dangerous Motherhood: Insanity and Childbirth in Victorian Britain.* (Compelling historical examples of postpartum psychosis.)

ON POSTPARTUM MOOD DISORDERS, INCLUDING PSYCHOSIS

Layperson oriented

Bennett, Shoshana S., and Pec Indman. *Beyond the Blues: A Guide to Understanding and Treating Prenatal and Postpartum Depression.* (Short, comprehensive, basic handbook; appendix has explanations/descriptions of medical terms and healthcare providers. One of my "top 5.")

Bennett, Shoshana S. *Postpartum Depression for Dummies.* (Excellent, easy-to-use reference on the full spectrum of postpartum mood disorders. One of my "top 5.")

Dix, Carol. *The New Mother Syndrome: Coping with Postpartum Stress and Depression.* (Wonderful list of resources. Almost a "top 5" but a little too out-of-date. Currently out of print.)

Dunnewold, Ann, and Diane G. Sanford. *Postpartum Survival Guide.* (Valuable resource for layperson and practitioner, packed with practical information.)

Poulin, Sandra. *The Mother-to-Mother Postpartum Depression Support Book.* (Illustrates full spectrum of postpartum mood disorders using first-person stories. Resource book list includes categories on recovery, biography, inspiration, comedic relief, and others.)

Puryear, Lucy J. *Understanding Your Moods When You're Expecting: Emotions, Mental Health, and Happiness—Before, During, and After Pregnancy.* (Planning for and coping with emotions throughout the pregnancy and postpartum experience. Excellent resource. Puryear's Web site at http://www.lucypuryear.com/resources also has good information/resources.)

Sichel, Deborah, and Jeanne Watson Driscoll. *Women's Moods: What Every Woman Must Know About Hormones, the Brain, and Emotional Health.* (Covers the lifespan of reproductive mental health. For every woman who wants to understand her brain. One of my "top 5.")

Practitioner and researcher oriented

Dunnewold, Ann L. *Evaluation and Treatment of Postpartum Emotional Disorders.*

Hamilton, James Alexander, and Patricia Neel Harberger, eds. *Postpartum Psychiatric Illness: A Picture Puzzle.* (Excellent resource covering issues ranging from endocrinology to medical insurance and law. One of my "top 5." Currently out of print.)

ON MEDICATION AND BREASTFEEDING

Bennett, Shoshana. *Pregnant on Prozac.* (Scheduled for release in January of 2009.)

Hale, Thomas W. *Medications and Mother's Milk: A Manual of Lactational Pharmacology*, 13th ed.

ON INFANTICIDE

Meyer, Cheryl L. , and Michelle Oberman. *Mothers Who Kill Their Children.*

Spencer, Suzy. *Breaking Point.* (Coverage of the Andrea Yates story.)

Spinelli, Margaret. *Infanticide: Psychosocial and Legal Perspectives on Mothers Who Kill.* (Wonderfully informative far beyond "infanticide." One of my "top 5.")

OTHER

Finn, Kristin K. *Bipolar and Pregnant: How to Manage and Succeed in Planning and Parenting while Living with Manic Depression.*

Riklan, David, and Dr. Joseph Cilea. *101 Great Ways to Improve Your Health.* (See #73 "Postpartum Emotional Health" by Cheryl Jazzar, MHR.)

Taylor, Verta. *Rock-A-By Baby: Feminism, Self-Help, and Postpartum Depression.*

Wolf, Naomi. *Misconceptions: Truth, Lies, and the Unexpected on the Journey to Motherhood.* (Contains extensive listing of organizations concerned with childbirth.)

ORGANIZATIONS AND ONLINE SOURCES OF INFORMATION

The Melanie Stokes Foundation
http://www.melaniesbattle.org
Melanie's story is in this book. This Web site was created by her mother to raise aware-
   ness after Melanie died. Visitors to the site can view and write in the Guestbook.

Katherine Stone's Web Log: Postpartum Progress
http://www.postpartumprogress.typepad.com
Peer support, breaking news, insightful commentary, advocacy and resources.

Massachusetts General Hospital Women's Center
http://www.womensmentalhealth.org
"Reproductive psychiatry resource and information center."

The Marcé Society
http://www.marcesociety.com
"An international society for the understanding, prevention and treatment of mental
   illness related to childbearing."

Medline
http://www.nlm.nih.gov/medlineplus/postpartumdepression.html
From the National Libraries of Medicine.

Jenny's Light
http://www.jennyslight.org
"A foundation to spread awareness & help support women and families dealing with
   postpartum illnesses." Jenny and her son Graham lost their lives due to postpar-
   tum mental illness.

MedEdPPD, "Mothers & Others"
http://www.mededppd.org
Created with the support of the National Institute for Mental Health to provide infor-
   mation on postpartum mood disorders.

"I'm Listening": Jane Honikman's Web site
http://www.janehonikman.com
Jane Honikman is the "mother" of PSI and an advocate for social support. Honik-
   man has also written two books for those interested in helping those with
   PPMDs, I'm Listening *and* Step by Step *(both are available through her*
   Web site). Honikman is the author of the "Universal message" of Postpartum
   Support International—"You are not alone, you are not to blame, there is help
   and you will be well."

Using Clinical Nutrition for Maternal Mental Health
http://www.wellpostpartum.com
A blog on clinical nutrition as prevention and treatment of perinatal mood disorders.

BabyCenter.com
http://www.babycenter.com
This is not a Web site dedicated to postpartum mood disorders—but it does contain
   good information, and it is where I first learned the name of this illness.

My Web site: Postpartum Experience
http://www.postpartumexperience.com
Lists additional resources.

RECOMMENDED BY SHOSHANA BENNETT

Motherrisk.org
http://www.motherrisk.org
Provides links and a search tool for a number of pregnancy-related topics.

ClearSky
http://www.clearsky-inc.com
"Finding and keeping joy," Dr. Shoshana Bennett's perinatal depression Web site.

Center for Complementary and Alternative Medicine
http://www.nccam.nih.gov
"Expanding horizons of healthcare" by National Institutes of Health.

Appendix B: Resources for Help

SUICIDE PREVENTION

National Hopeline Network:
1-800-SUICIDE (1-800-784-2433)
http://www.hopeline.com

National Suicide Prevention Lifeline:
1-800-273-TALK (1-800-273-8255)
http://www.suicidedpreventionlifeline.org

ORGANIZATIONS FOR THOSE WITH POSTPARTUM MOOD DISORDERS

Postpartum Support International:
PSI Postpartum Depression Help Line: 1-800-944-4PPD (4773)
http://www.postpartum.net
Peer support network, wide variety of information for laypersons, researchers, and practitioners. Quarterly newsletter and annual conference. PSI coordinators are volunteers who can assist in finding a variety of resources. The PSI Web site has a search function to find a coordinator in your state or geographic area. PSI itself is a volunteer organization offering assistance and is not a provider of, or substitute for, medical care.
For Spanish speakers, from the PSI Web site:
APOYO DE PSI PARA LAS FAMILIAS HISPANO PARLANTES
1-800-944-4773 #1
Llame al número de teléfono gratuito para obtener recursos, apoyo e información gratuita.
Déjenos un mensaje y un voluntario le devolverá la llamada.

Podrá encontrar más información y recursos en la página web de PSI. Presione en el botón siguiente.
In English this translates to: Call the toll-free phoneline, select #1, for resources, support, and information.
Leave us a message, and one of our support volunteers will call you back.
We also have Online Resources on the PSI Web site.
Telephone: 1-800-944-4773, #1

The Online PPD Support Group:
http://www.ppdsupportpage.com
Online PPD support group featuring live chats, posting boards, chat rooms, email forums and links. Online coordinator is Jessica Banas.

Fathers' Coordinators and Web site:
http://www.postpartumdads.org
Intended to help dads and families by providing information and guidance.

Ruth Rhoden Craven Foundation:
http://www.ppdsupport.org
Named after Ruth Craven, who died when her son was two and a half months old. The foundation's goal is to provide information and support ... and to serve as a resource to those in the medical community.

Postpartum Resource Center of New York:
http://www.postpartumny.org
One of the first organizations to provide state-specific and general information and support to women with PPMDs. (More organizations are listed on my Web site: www.postpartumexperience.com)

The Center for Postpartum Health:
http://www.postpartumhealth.com
"Where mothers are mothered" Emphasizes assessment and prevention.

Solace for Mothers: Healing after Traumatic Childbirth:
http://www.solaceformothers.org
Online community with resources for those dealing with recovery from challenging or traumatic childbirth experience. Also has a warmline: 877-SOLACE.

OTHER ORGANIZATIONS

NAMI: National Alliance on Mental Illness:
http://www.nami.org
Dedicated to the eradication of mental illness and improvement of quality of life for those affected.

DBSA: Depression and Bipolar Support Alliance:
http://www.dbsalliance.org
"Improving the lives of people living with mood disorders."

NASPOG: North American Society for Psychosocial Obstetrics and Gynecology:
http://www.naspog.org
Purpose is "to foster scholarly scientific and clinical study of the biopsychosocial aspects of obstetric and gynecologic medicine."

Index

abusive relationships, 37, 70, 146; child abuse and, 61, 80; in stories, 106, 140–44

Advancing American Priorities Act, 64

ALI (American Law Institute), 56

alternative and complementary medicine practitioners, 19–20, 115–16. *See also* Center for Complementary and Alternative Medicine; diet; vitamins

American College of Obstetricians and Gynecologists, 63

American Law Institute, 56

American Medical Association, 31

American Psychiatric Association, 25

America's Women: 400 years of Dolls, Drudges, Helpmates and Heroines, 30

anger, 57, 72–73, 80–81, 137; and depression, 4; as symptom, 9, 17, 69; toward husband, 71, 75, 79; toward mother, 84

antidepressant, causing manic episode, 5, 146

antipsychotic, 16–17

anxiety, postpartum, 3, 4, 13, 16; and OCD, 7–8; in stories, 93, 111, 116–20, 135, 140

appetite, 4, 132

Are You There Alone?, 31

assessment, 10, 13, 82; and prevention, 148, 164; responsibility for, xix. *See also* screening

attorneys, xx, 58–62, 64–65, 149

awareness, 26–28, 57; 64, 148–49

baby blues, 3, 10, 38–39, 48; in stories, 70, 90, 117, 140

behavior, x, 2, 16, 37, 61–62; ability to control, 55; help-seeking, 28, 48; that illustrates delusional themes, 32–33; normal postpartum, xvi, 57; unlike former self, 35, 60; violent and inappropriate, 32

beliefs: common, xvii; delusional, 43, 62, 121; false, 9, 16

Bennett, Shoshana, 1, 3, 15, 24, 159–62

bipolar disorder: and DSM classification, 25, 48; connection between PPP and, xix, 12, 20, 29, 146, 148; in stories, 80–81, 84, 112, 118; misdiagnois of, 5; postpartum described, 4; spectrum, 29; support alliance, 165; treatment of, 20–21

blame, 28, 35–37, 43–45; in stories, 69, 75–76, 96; PSI universal message on, xxv, 9, 27, 150, 161

Blocker, Carol, 29, 131, 136–37; and MOTHERS Act, 63–64; letters to, 137

blood loss, 71–72

About the Author and Contributors

TERESA M. TWOMEY, JD is Co-Coordinator for Postpartum Support International in Connecticut. She served earlier as Coordinator for Postpartum Support International in Virginia, and as a Public Reviewer for the National Institute of Mental Health. Twomey, who has been a faculty member at Longwood University in Virginia, and a Paralegal Instructor of Master Technical Institute in New Jersey, practiced law and professional mediation before experiencing postpartum psychosis herself. After her recovery, she put her law career on hold to become an advocate for women with postpartum mood disorders.

SHOSHANA BENNETT, PHD, contributed the first two chapters: 1. More than Depression (explaining the differences among Postpartum Psychosis, Postpartum Depression, and Postpartum Obsessive-Compulsive Disorder) and 2. Psychological Views. Bennett is a past president of Postpartum Support International and the founder and director of Postpartum Assistance for Mothers. She is also an author of *Postpartum Depression for Dummies* and *Pregnant on Prozac*, plus the co-author of *Beyond the Blues: A Guide to Understanding and Treating Prenatal and Postpartum Depression*.

The first-person stories were contributed by women who have suffered this illness, and who want to help other women who had or have postpartum psychosis know that they are not alone and will be well.

Carol Blocker provided her story of her daughter Melanie's illness. Blocker is a staunch advocate for those with this illness and is a driving force behind the legislation currently being considered by the federal legislature.

Katherine provided her story of infanticide and incarceration. In spite of her bizarre behavior, she was sent home to care for her newborn. Her story illustrates how little is often done for women with this illness, even when it is obvious, and the predictable tragedy that results.